Diabetes Nutrition Q&A For Health Professionals

Joyce Green Pastors, RD, MS, CDE, Editor
Marilynn S. Arnold, MS, RD, CDE
Anne Daly, MS, RD, BC-ADM, CDE
Marion Franz, MS, RD, CDE
Hope S. Warshaw, MMSc, RD, CDE

American Diabetes Association.
Cure • Care • Commitment®

Director, Book Publishing, John Fedor; *Associate Director, Professional Books,* Christine B. Charlip; *Editor,* Joyce Raynor; *Associate Director, Book Production,* Peggy M. Rote; *Composition,* Circle Graphics, Inc.; *Cover Design,* Mac Designs; *Printer,* Port City Press

Printed in the United States of America
1 3 5 7 9 10 8 6 4 2

⊚ The paper in this publication meets the requirements of the ANSI Standard Z39.48-1992 (permanence of paper).

ADA titles may be purchased for business or promotional use or for special sales. To purchase this book in large quantities, or for custom editions of this book with your logo, contact Lee Romano Sequeira, Special Sales & Promotions, at the address below, or at LRomano@diabetes.org or call 703-299-2046.

American Diabetes Association
1701 North Beauregard Street
Alexandria, Virginia 22311

Library of Congress Cataloging-in-Publication Data

Diabetes nutrition Q & A for health professionals / Joyce Green Pastors ... [et al.].
    p. ; cm.
  Includes bibliographical references and index.
  ISBN 1-58040-199-6 (pbk. : alk. paper)
1. Diabetes—Nutritional aspects—Miscellanea. I. Title: Diabetes nutrition Q and A for health professionals. II. Pastors, Joyce Green.
[DNLM: 1. Diabetes Mellitus—diet therapy. 2. Diabetic Diet. 3. Nutrition—physiology. 4. Patient Education. WK 818 D536 2003]
RC662.D525 2003
616.4'620654—dc22

                                   2003063006

CONTENTS

PROTEIN

FAT

Medication

Pattern Management

Obesity/Weight Maintenance

Special Populations

OLDER PEOPLE

GESTATIONAL DIABETES

Common Concerns/Issues

EATING AWAY FROM HOME

HYPOGLYCEMIA/HYPERGLYCEMIA/SICK DAYS

PORTION CONTROL

NUTRITION LABEL

SNACKING

Prevention of Diabetes

Resources

DIETITIAN ACCESS/REFERRAL

EDUCATIONAL RESOURCES

REIMBURSEMENT

FOREWORD

Nutrition is a hallmark of treatment in diabetes mellitus. This is true irrespective of the type of diabetes a person has. Nevertheless, nutrition advice given by health professionals to patients is often inadequate. This is partly due to a lack of time on the part of the professional, but also often to a lack of appropriate knowledge. This book tries to correct for the latter. It is a clearly written, informative, and practical guide for the health professional.

Diabetes brings with it countless questions that a patient would like to have answered. These deal with total calories, macronutrient proportions, specific fats, specific carbohydrates, quantity and quality of protein, energy requirements, caloric and noncaloric sweeteners, glycemic index, carbohydrate counting, alcohol, dietary supplements, sodium needs, meal planning, physical activity, interactions between medications and food, and snacking. The patients also have concerns with regard to life cycle issues: childhood, adolescence, pregnancy, and old age. They are increasingly worried about eating outside the home, because restaurant meals have grown greatly in terms of portion sizes served and calorie content over the last two decades and because eating out has become a common, in some cases everyday, occurrence. They have a need to know more about referrals to dietitians, educational resources, and reimbursement, issues that are extremely important to patients but for which they often get very little advice.

Diabetes Nutrition Q&A for Health Professionals addresses these issues in a simple and straightforward manner. Its format allows the busy practitioner to focus in on particular questions in an efficient manner. The authors have been careful to present their answers in an evidence-based fashion that gives credibility to their treatment of the issues.

The prevalence of diabetes mellitus is growing at a rapid pace in this country and throughout the world. There are millions and millions of people with diabetes, who require lifelong education, counseling, and understanding. The more patients comprehend their disease and how to manage it, the more likely they will be to control it well and prevent its devastating complications. Health professionals have a great responsibility to help them with this. Over the last three decades, there has been a growing emphasis on the importance of a team approach to diabetes care. The doctor, the nurse, the dietitian, the educator, the exercise expert, the pharmacist, the psychologist, the podiatrist, and other necessary specialists all work together with and on behalf of patients. For these health professionals to do their job well, they have to be adequately prepared. The information in *Diabetes Nutrition Q&A* is enormously helpful in this regard—it provides a sound basis from which to provide nutrition counseling.

I hope that this book can be translated into many other languages and widely disseminated. Information is power—power to understand, to modify behavior, to improve control, to reduce the risk of complications, and to enhance the quality of life.

Xavier Pi-Sunyer, MD, MPH
Professor of Medicine, Columbia University College
of Physicians and Surgeons
Chief, Division of Endocrinology, Diabetes, and Nutrition
Director, New York Obesity Research Center

ABOUT THE AUTHORS

Joyce Green Pastors, RD, MS, CDE, is a Diabetes Nutrition Specialist with the Virginia Center for Diabetes Professional Education and an Assistant Professor of Medical Education in Internal Medicine, Division of Endocrinology, University of Virginia Health System. She is a past chair of the Diabetes Care and Education Practice Group of the American Dietetic Association. She has also coauthored several publications of the American Diabetes Association and the American Dietetic Association, most notably, *Facilitating Lifestyle Change: A Resource Manual* and *Diabetes Medical Nutrition Therapy: A Professional Guide to Management and Nutrition Education Resources.*

Marilynn S. Arnold, MS, RD, CDE, is a second-career dietitian whose 14 years in diabetes has been divided between the academic and the practical. As a nutrition specialist for the Michigan Diabetes Research and Training Center for 8 years, she participated in translation research and contributed to several publications, including *Life with Diabetes*, published by the ADA. She continues to explore her interest in facilitating behavior change and providing MNT in a nurse-dietitian private practice.

Anne Daly, MS, RD, BC-ADM, CDE, is an award-winning dietitian and certified diabetes educator with 25 years of experience specializing in diabetes care. She is the Director of Nutrition and Diabetes Education at the Springfield Diabetes and Endocrine Center in Springfield, Illinois, and a Past President, Health Care &

Education, of the American Diabetes Association, and a nationally recognized author and speaker, with special interest in obesity treatment and diabetes prevention. Anne is a coauthor of *101 Weight Loss Tips for Preventing and Controlling Diabetes*, published by ADA.

Marion J. Franz, MS, RD, CDE, was the Director of Nutrition and Professional Education at the International Diabetes Center in Minneapolis for over 20 years and is now an independent nutrition/health consultant. She led the task forces that wrote the American Diabetes Association's diabetes nutrition recommendations in 1994 and 2002 and edited the 4th and 5th editions of *A CORE Curriculum for Diabetes Educators* for the American Association of Diabetes Educators. Marion coauthored the ADA book *Implementing Group and Individual Medical Nutrition Therapy for Diabetes*.

Hope S. Warshaw, MMSc, RD, CDE, has been a diabetes educator nearly 25 years. She owns Hope Warshaw Associates, in Alexandria, Virginia, providing individual nutrition and diabetes counseling and pump training to people with diabetes, consulting with companies manufacturing diabetes and nutrition-related products, and writing for diabetes publications. Hope is the author of several books published by ADA, including *Diabetes Meal Planning Made Easy* and *The Guide to Healthy Restaurant Eating*, and is the coauthor of *Complete Guide to Carb Counting*.

INTRODUCTION

For most people who develop diabetes, food and eating become of primary concern. What should I eat now? How can I lose weight? These are questions any health care professional is likely to hear from a diabetes patient. Diabetes, perhaps more than any other chronic disease, is full of myths and misinformation concerning nutrition. To help our patients sort truth from rumor when they come to us for advice about diabetes nutrition, we need to understand the facts.

Diabetes Nutrition Q&A for Health Professionals provides answers to the questions commonly asked by patients, as well as our colleagues, about nutrition and diabetes. Here you will find exactly the information that busy practitioners, who don't have the time to go to the literature on specific topics, are looking for, backed by evidence-based research and including references and resources, when indicated. In addition, the answers reflect the best clinical judgments, expertise, and practices of each of the authors—all dietitians and diabetes educators with many years of experience in nutrition and diabetes education.

We asked the most pertinent and charged questions, many controversial in diabetes nutrition, and provided answers that stand up to scrutiny. Vital topics include medical nutrition therapy, physical activity, medications, obesity and weight management, prevention of diabetes, resources for patients, reimbursement, and more. Have you ever wondered *why* we make some of the recommendations that we do? Here you will find the evidence on whether some carbohydrates are better than others, whether patients need fish oil supplements, whether eating low–glycemic index foods will improve control, and whether antioxidant supplements are beneficial.

We also help you teach patients to be more physically active and the truth about high-protein–low-carbohydrate diets, and help clarify issues such as preventing obesity in children, insurance reimbursement to treat obesity, and basic and advanced carbohydrate counting. And there is so much more. In fact, this book began as a book of "101 tips," but in the process of generating ideas for questions, writing the answers, and reviewing the final drafts, it was evident that this was an opportunity to explain the science that supports the way we practice. We hope you find this book useful in your practice working with diabetes patients.

On a personal note, I would like to acknowledge my colleagues and coauthors, Lynn Arnold, Anne Daly, Marion Franz, and Hope Warshaw. This book is more comprehensive, in-depth, and practical because of their expertise. We all learned and benefited greatly from working together and sharing our knowledge and experiences.

In addition, I would like to acknowledge my long-time colleague and professional partner at the University of Virginia Diabetes Center, Terry Saunders, PhD. I appreciate his flexibility in allowing me the time to work on this project and his understanding of the importance of opportunities such as these to enhance professional growth.

Joyce Green Pastors, RD, MS, CDE
Editor

Medical Nutrition Therapy Goals

What are the primary medical nutrition therapy (MNT) goals for people with type 1 and type 2 diabetes?

The primary goal of diabetes MNT is to help people with diabetes attain and maintain optimal metabolic outcomes for glucose, lipids, and blood pressure (1,2).

For type 1 diabetes, the primary goal is to establish a reasonable and achievable eating plan that can be used to integrate a desired insulin regimen. Shortly after the diagnosis and after the patient has settled into the day-to-day management of diabetes, present each individual/family with the range of insulin regimens available today. Encourage people with type 1 diabetes to choose a diabetes management plan that matches well with all facets of their lifestyle and desired level of sophistication and intensification.

For type 2 diabetes, the goal is to identify behavior changes/lifestyle interventions that can help individuals achieve optimal metabolic outcomes for glucose, lipids, and blood pressure. Health care professionals can assist people with diabetes in identifying several small changes that they can make in their eating habits and physical activity level. Over time, these small changes accumulate and can lead to the desired outcomes. Encourage all people with diabetes to identify changes that they are willing and able to make and to make the easiest ones first. Initial success can provide positive reinforcement to continue.

Today, people in a wide range of age groups and stages of life are affected by diabetes. Contrary to older definitions of who develops type 1 and type 2 diabetes, now more adults over 30 years of age develop type 1 diabetes and more children and adolescents develop type 2 diabetes. The type of diabetes, age, lifestyle, stage of life, other medical concerns, and possibly diabetes complications also must be considered in setting MNT goals.

Another essential element of all diabetes MNT is sufficient and consistent education and support. It has been well documented in the Diabetes Control and Complications Trial, the Diabetes Prevention Program, and other long-term trials that for people to make the difficult behavior changes required in diabetes management they need both initial and continuing education and support. Clearly, a one-time "diet instruction" does not help people make the changes necessary to achieve positive metabolic outcomes.

Which MNT goal is likely to be affected first by lifestyle interventions?

The first goal of MNT is to help people with diabetes attain and maintain blood glucose levels as close to normal as is safely possible. As reported in numerous studies such as the United Kingdom Prospective Diabetes Study (3) and the nutrition practice guidelines clinical trials (4,5), changes in food/nutrition generally improve glycemia almost immediately. In type 2 diabetes, this acute improvement is attributed to a reduction in energy intake. In type 1 diabetes, the improvement is ascribed to a better match between insulin regimens and food/carbohydrate intake.

Because the effect of MNT is observed first on glycemia, many dietitians initially focus on carbohydrate counting—helping individuals with diabetes understand what foods contain carbohydrate, what are average portion sizes, and how many carbohydrate servings to select for meals. This approach also provides guidelines to assist the person with diabetes who needs to eat less.

Changes in food choices and carbohydrate intake will also improve lipids and lower blood pressure, but it may take longer to see the benefits. At follow-up visits with the dietitian, lifestyle interventions for improving lipids (such as lowering saturated fat and dietary cholesterol) and for lowering blood pressure can be addressed.

What is a "healthy diet"?

A plan of eating that promotes health and well-being and reduces risk for many chronic diseases requires multiple foods and nutrients. A healthy eating plan consists of

- five or more servings per day from a variety of fruits and vegetables
- six or more servings per day of grain products, including whole grain foods
- two or three servings of fish per week
- two servings per day of low-fat dairy products
- limited servings of lean meat or poultry
- minimal or healthy fat choices

Just taking a supplement to replace nutrients in foods isn't the answer because it is unknown what it is in foods that cause them to be healthy. Most research attempting to answer the question, "What is a 'healthy diet'?" has focused on individual nutrients such as fats or carbohydrates, or on certain vitamins or minerals, or on individual foods or components of food such as fiber, sucrose, fructose, or nonnutritive sweeteners. This is because a basic principle of research is to design studies that have only one variable so it can be determined whether that variable has an effect. However, this type of research hasn't really provided answers about what is a "healthy diet" and what are healthy foods. Recent research suggests that no single nutrient or food by itself is the answer. Instead, health benefits are realized from food patterns that include combinations of foods containing multiple nutrients and nonnutrients. An example of this approach is the Dietary Approach to Stop Hypertension study (6). Food patterns identified in this study were five to seven servings of fruits and vegetables and two servings of nonfat dairy products eaten in the context of a diet that also contained minimal servings of meats and fats. Other studies have supported this approach (7,8).

Focusing on patterns, rather than single foods or nutrients, makes research attempting to determine the mechanisms through which components of the eating plan affect a health outcome difficult. However, it is a practical approach to making realistic nutrition recommendations for improving health. The American Heart Association (AHA) guidelines 2001 are another example of this approach (9). AHA guidelines are presented in terms of foods and food servings and not in terms of single macronutrients or other food components.

The American Diabetes Association 2002 nutrition recommendations address specific food and nutrition issues for the prevention or treatment of diabetes and do not attempt to define a "healthy diet." Instead they support and incorporate nutrition recommendations from other major organizations such as the US Department of Agriculture (*Dietary Guidelines for Americans*) (10), the AHA, the National Cholesterol Education Program Adult Treatment Panel III (11), and the 7th Report of the Joint National Committee on Prevention, Detection, Evaluation, and Treatment of High Blood Pressure (12). For people with diabetes to eat healthfully, choosing a variety of foods from the food patterns listed above is what it is all about.

Medical Nutrition Therapy Outcomes

What are the expected outcomes from MNT on glycated hemoglobin A1C (A1C) and fasting plasma glucose, and when should they be evaluated?

Randomized controlled trials, observational studies, and meta-analysis indicate that MNT improves metabolic outcomes such as blood glucose and A1C in people with diabetes (13,14). The evidence also supports the need for ongoing evaluation and intervention to achieve clinical goals and outcomes.

Specifically, the randomized controlled trials and observational studies of diabetes MNT have demonstrated an expected decrease in A1C outcomes of ~1–2% (a 15–24% decrease) and a 50- to 100-mg/dl decrease in fasting plasma glucose concentrations. In people newly diagnosed with type 2 diabetes, the United Kingdom Prospective Diabetes Study (3) and the Nutrition Practice Guidelines (NPG) for type 2 diabetes clinical trial (4) reported an average decrease in A1C of 2% from intensive nutrition therapy provided by dietitians. In people with type 2 diabetes of an average duration of 4 years, the NPG trial reported an average decrease of A1C of 1% due to intensive therapy provided by dietitians who followed the NPG.

In people newly diagnosed with type 1 diabetes, a clinical trial using the NPG for type 1 diabetes reported an average decrease in A1C of 1% from intensive nutrition therapy provided by dietitians who followed the NPG (5). The Dose Adjusted for Normal Eating trial conducted in Great Britain reported a 1% decrease in A1C in patients with type 1 diabetes who were instructed by dietitians on how to adjust mealtime insulin based on the carbohydrate content of meals (15).

This evidence suggests that medical nutrition therapy has the greatest impact at initial diagnosis, but continues to be effective at any time during the disease process. The glycemic outcomes from MNT are similar to those from many oral glucose-lowering medications.

In people with type 2 diabetes, the effects of MNT on A1C are evident by 6 weeks to 3 months, at which time the dietitian should assess whether therapy goals have been met by changes in lifestyle or whether additions or changes in medications are needed (4). At ~6 weeks after the initial nutrition consult, the dietitian needs to determine whether the individual is making progress toward their personal goals. If no progress is evident, consider revising the nutrition care plan. At 3 months, changes in medical therapy are recommended if:

- blood glucose concentrations or A1C percentages have not shown a downward trend
- the person has lost weight with no improvement in glucose
- the person is doing well with the nutrition and physical activity goals but further nutrition interventions are unlikely to improve medical outcomes
- the person has done all that she or he can or is willing to do

This is the time to consider additions or changes in medication(s).

What are the expected outcomes on lipids and hypertension from MNT, and when should they be evaluated?

Cardiovascular disease is the primary cause of mortality and morbidity in people with diabetes. Optimal lipid concentrations and blood pressure reduce the risk of cardiovascular disease, and MNT plays a major role in achieving those metabolic goals. Evidence as to the expected outcomes for MNT specific to people with diabetes is not available, and therefore, evidence from clinical studies in nondiabetic subjects (16) must be used to extrapolate expected outcomes for people with diabetes. A meta-analysis of 37 nutrition intervention studies in nondiabetic free-living subjects in which saturated fats were restricted to 7–10% of energy intake and dietary cholesterol to 200–300 mg daily, resulted in a 10–13% (24–32 mg/dl) decrease in plasma total cholesterol, 12–16% (19–25 mg/dl) decrease in low-density lipoprotein (LDL) cholesterol, and 8% (15–17 mg/dl) decrease in triglycerides (17).

The American Diabetes Association recommends that, for people with diabetes, the goal for LDL cholesterol is <100 mg/dl (18). If the LDL cholesterol exceeds the goal by >25 mg/dl, American Diabetes Association recommends that pharmacological therapy be started at the same time as MNT for people at high-risk (i.e., those with prior myocardial infarction and/or other cardiovascular risk factors). In other people with diabetes, MNT is initially used as monotherapy and may be evaluated at the 6-week interval, with consideration of pharmacological therapy between 3 and 6 months.

A meta-analysis in nondiabetic subjects in which moderate reductions in sodium intake (2,400 mg/day) were employed was associated with declines in systolic and diastolic blood pressures of 6 and 2 mmHg in people with hypertension and of 3 and 1 mmHg in people who were normotensive (19). Although there are wide variations in blood pressure responses, the lower the sodium intake, the lower the blood pressure (20). Responses to sodium reduction may be greater in subjects who are "salt sensitive," a characteristic of many people with diabetes. Clinical trial data suggest that a weight loss of 4.5 kg (10 lb) can be as effective as first-level drugs in controlling blood pressure (6). A low-fat eating plan that includes fruits and vegetables and low-fat dairy products (e.g., Dietary Approach to Stop Hypertension diet) also reduces blood pressure (21). Blood pressure should be measured at every medical visit.

Nutrient Recommendations

CARBOHYDRATE

How much carbohydrate does a person with diabetes really need?

The amount of carbohydrate that will best help individuals with diabetes meet their clinical goals will vary. The Recommended Dietary Allowance (RDA) for the general population is 130 g carbohydrate/day. The RDAs are set to meet the needs of most (97–98%) people in a group and may be used by individuals as a target intake. However, the actual carbohydrate intake in the United States is much higher (partly to meet calorie needs), with a median intake of 200–330 g/day for men and 180–230 for women (22).

Carbohydrate is an essential nutrient and the body's preferred fuel. As stated by the Institute of Medicine:

> *The primary role of carbohydrate is to provide energy to cells in the body, particularly the brain, which is the only carbohydrate-dependent organ in the body. The Recommended Dietary Allowance for carbohydrate is set at 130 g/day for adults and children based on the minimum amount of glucose utilized by the brain (22).*

People with diabetes can use the RDA as a starting point. If distributed equally between three meals, this would mean targeting about 45 g carbohydrate per meal. If, as outlined in the nutrition recommendations (2), protein intake is 15–20% of the total calories, saturated fat is <10%, and polyunsaturated fat is ~10%, then 60–70% of the calories remain to come from carbohydrate and monounsaturated fat. Typically, 45–50% of total energy comes from carbohydrate. In general, this translates into 45–75 g per meal for women and 60–90 g per meal for men.

Because carbohydrate most affects short-term glucose response, people with diabetes may get the message to eat as little carbohydrate as possible to help control glucose levels. Some may replace their carbohydrate intake with protein. However, much of the foods we eat as protein (e.g., meat, eggs, cheese) contain saturated fat. Fat—especially saturated fat—appears to increase insulin resistance, which, in turn, affects glucose control (2) (see page 34).

Foods high in carbohydrate, such as grains, fruits, and milk, provide nutrients necessary to maintain health. Although carbohydrate from a handful of jellybeans and three slices of whole wheat bread are both digested and metabolized to about the same amount of glucose, the vitamins, minerals, fiber, and satiety offered are not.

For individuals with diabetes, specific carbohydrate recommendations are based on an assessment of their current eating habits, metabolic profile, and treatment goals. Consideration is given to the balance between carbohydrate, protein, and fat. People with diabetes require all the macronutrients, just as people in general do.

Are sugars a "fast-acting carbohydrate"?

No. All carbohydrate-containing foods raise blood glucose levels in nearly identical rates, and therefore there are no "fast-acting carbohydrates." For years, the most commonly given advice to people with diabetes about what to eat was to avoid "simple" or "fast-acting sugars" because they were small molecules that would be rapidly digested and absorbed into the bloodstream, causing glucose levels to rise higher than "complex carbohydrates" would. The problem with this statement has to do with terminology. When referring to the carbohydrates commonly found in foods, the following terms are preferred: sugars and starches. This classification is based on the recommendations of the Food and Agriculture Organization of the

United Nations and the World Health Organization (23) and the Dietary Reference Intakes (22). Terms such as "simple sugars," "fast-acting carbohydrates," and "complex carbohydrates" cannot be defined based on chemical structure (i.e., degree of polymerization). In other words, these terms were "made up" for the general public, and thus, use of these terms is not recommended.

It is still often assumed that sugars and juices are "fast-acting" carbohydrates and, therefore, should be avoided. However, it turns out that foods rich in sugars such as milk and fruits tend to have lower glycemic index values than most common starches (24). Common sugars are ~50% glucose and 50% fructose or lactose (i.e., galactose). Fructose and galactose produce lower glucose responses than glucose because they are primarily stored in the liver as glycogen and, thus, do not enter the general circulation. Starches are polymers of glucose and are, therefore, 100% glucose.

In early research studies on glycemic responses to different carbohydrates, the effects of 50 g carbohydrate from dextrose (a sugar) and different starches were compared. Although the peak responses from different carbohydrates occurred at approximately the same time, there were differences in the height of the glucose peak (25). That is, some carbohydrates cause the glucose peak response to be higher but not at a faster rate. For example, the peak glucose response is higher for glucose compared to rice, bread, corn, or potatoes, but the peak response occurs at approximately the same time. Additional studies in subjects with type 1 or type 2 diabetes and in subjects without diabetes compared 42 g glucose to fructose, sucrose, and potato or wheat starch. Again, although fructose produced the lowest glycemic response, absorption rates and peak increments were the same (26).

The implication of these studies in regard to the treatment of hypoglycemia is that glucose and starch should probably be recommended over orange juice and milk.

The problems with recommending starch are primarily the issues of easy access, portability, and spoilage (e.g., crackers crumble and bread, rice, and potatoes aren't usually accessible and easily become moldy). Therefore, 100% glucose tablets or gel would be the best choice.

Even though all carbohydrates raise blood glucose levels in nearly identical rates, the advice to be careful of sugars is still good advice—provided it is given for the correct reason. Often, foods that contain sugars are high in total carbohydrate as well as fat and calories, such as soft drinks and desserts. When people with diabetes limit added sugars, it may help control blood glucose levels. But if they choose to enjoy a sweet or dessert—as does nearly everyone once in awhile—teach them to substitute the sweet for another carbohydrate in their food/meal plan. If a person is able to adjust their medication, such as insulin or an oral glucose–lowering medication, they can cover additional carbohydrate from sweets with medication (1,2).

Are some foods that contain carbohydrate better for people with diabetes than others?

Today, there is much contradictory and confusing advice concerning the role of carbohydrate in meal plans for people with diabetes. There are two points to keep in mind when answering this question. The first point is that foods containing carbohydrates known to be part of a healthy eating plan—fruits, vegetables, grains, and low-fat dairy products—are always better choices than foods that do not contribute to health, such as soft drinks, sweets, snack chips and crackers, desserts, and so on.

But, do some foods that contain carbohydrate raise glucose levels more than others and therefore require more insulin? Research has shown that a number of factors determine the individual effects of foods containing 50 g carbohydrates on postprandial glucose levels (27). However, what happens when a variety of foods in more usual portion sizes and containing carbohydrate are eaten at meals or for snacks? There are now ~20 studies documenting that when people with type 1 or type 2 diabetes choose a variety of starchy foods or a variety of starchy foods and sucrose-containing foods and keep the total amount of carbohydrate in the meal or snack the same, the blood glucose response is the same. Furthermore, similar amounts of insulin are needed to keep blood glucose in the normal range.

Therefore, the second point is that the total amount of carbohydrate eaten is more important than the source (starch or sugar) or type (high or low glycemic index) of foods. For a healthy eating plan, focus on the carbohydrate-containing foods rich in vitamins, minerals, and fiber, such as fruits, vegetables, grains, and low-fat dairy products.

Does a high-carbohydrate eating plan increase triglyceride levels?

It depends. In weight-maintenance diets that are either high in carbohydrate (carbohydrate >55% of total energy) or high in monounsaturated fats (total fat ~40% and monounsaturated fats ~25% of total energy, respectively), reductions in low-density lipoprotein cholesterol and improvements in fasting glucose concentrations are similar (28). However, the high-carbohydrate diet increased triglycerides by ~50 mg/dl and postmeal glycemia to a greater extent than the diet that replaced some of the carbohydrate with monounsaturated fats (28). In contrast, an energy-reduced diet that was low in fat and high in carbohydrate, compared to a diet that was high in monounsaturated fat, had no detrimental effect on triglycerides (29). The effect of a high percentage of carbohydrate on triglycerides, therefore, appears to be dependent on the total energy intake and the amount of carbohydrate.

There is no evidence that carbohydrates raise triglyceride levels in controlled research studies in which carbohydrate is <55% of total energy intake. And it is unlikely that people with type 2 diabetes will consume meals that are >55% of total energy from carbohydrate. For example, in the United Kingdom Prospective Diabetes Study, people newly diagnosed with type 2 diabetes received intensive nutrition counseling from dietitians for 3 months before being randomized into study groups. The intent of the intervention was to encourage individuals to eat 50–55% of their calories as carbohydrate and 30–35% of their calories from fat. Despite the intensive intervention, carbohydrate intake only increased to 43% of calories, and the fat intake decreased to 37% of calories (30). Percentages of macronutrients in the eating plans of people with type 2 diabetes in the US are similar.

An analysis of carbohydrate intake in US adults by the National Health and Nutrition Examination Study III showed that a higher percentage of carbohydrate (>57% in men and >59% in women) was also associated with a higher triglyceride concentrations and lower high-density lipoprotein (HDL) cholesterol. However, eating plans that were moderately high in carbohydrate (50–55% of energy) were associated with low cardiovascular risks and with favorable lipid profiles (i.e., lower cholesterol and triglyceride levels and higher HDL cholesterol levels) (31).

Therefore, a reduction in total energy intake, a moderate intake of carbohydrate (45–50% of calories), and a lower fat intake is the approach that is most likely to lead to improvement in lipids, including triglycerides. In general, low-fat eating plans that are moderate to high in carbohydrate (45–50%) are associated with a modest weight loss and decreases in triglycerides and cholesterol and increases in HDL cholesterol (32,33).

What is the glycemic index? Will eating low–glycemic index foods improve glucose control?

The glycemic index (GI) is a method for classifying carbohydrates based on their blood glucose response proposed by Jenkins et al. in 1981 (34). The GI is formally defined as the incremental area under the blood glucose curve (AUC) after the consumption of 50 g carbohydrate from a test food divided by the AUC after eating a similar amount of a control food, generally white bread or glucose (35). Because no factor limits the rate of digestion of polysaccharide into glucose, starchy foods do not necessarily have a lower GI than do simple sugars (36). In general, refined grain products and potatoes have a higher GI, legumes and unprocessed grains have a moderate GI, and nonstarchy fruit and vegetables have a lower GI.

The GI only measures glucose above the beginning fasting glucose level, and this has been a criticism of the test (37). If it were to measure what occurs naturally, fasting blood glucose levels would decrease over time, and the AUC would be greater. Several experts favor the use of the whole AUC as the real measure of glucose availability. If the AUC is calculated in this manner, the differences in GIs between foods are greatly attenuated. For example, a person with a fasting glucose of 75 mg/dl ingests two foods, one with a GI of 100 and the other a GI of 72. If the GI is calculated by using the whole glucose AUC instead of only the area above the fasting glucose, the values would be 100 and 92, respectively. The difference changes from 29 units to 8 units (37).

Another problem with the GI is that it uses a 2-h standard for when to end the test. People with diabetes, particularly type 2 diabetes, require longer than 2 h for their blood glucose concentrations to return to normal, if at all, because of the diminished or lost first phase insulin secretion response. Thus, the differences in GI also would be considerably less if the AUC was calculated for a more reasonable postprandial period of 4 h. Furthermore, the GI is measured in morning, after an overnight fast. Several studies have reported that if the GI is measured after lunch, the differences in GI would be considerably less than for breakfast. Individuals with diabetes are the most glucose intolerant in the morning due to circulating counterregulatory hormones. Glucose tolerance improves after eating breakfast.

All of these research results may offer reasons why the long-term improvement in glycemia from low-GI diets, compared to high-GI diets, has been controversial; a few studies report improvements in glycated hemoglobin A1C (A1C) or fructosamine, but most report no differences (27). Fourteen studies have compared diets with a low GI to diets with a high GI for at least 4 weeks. Two studies showed improvements in A1C, whereas eight studies reported no differences in A1C levels (27). Six studies reported improvements in fructosamine (i.e., a short-term measure of overall glucose control), whereas six studies showed no differences (not all studies measured both tests) (27). A meta-analysis reported a small improvement in A1C of ~0.4% from low versus high GI diets (38). Compared to other MNT interventions that have demonstrated a 1–2% decrease in A1C (13,14), this effect is modest at best (39).

There is not sufficient evidence of long-term benefit to recommend general use of the glycemic index in type 1 or type 2 patients with diabetes (37). Rather, the GI can be used as an adjunct to help "fine-tune" glycemic control. Some people may benefit from choosing low-GI foods, especially at breakfast, and others may not. Only by testing blood glucose levels pre- and postmeal will individuals be able to determine whether some foods raise their glucose levels more than others. However, for accuracy, the total amount of carbohydrate in the meals tested must be kept the same and blood glucose levels must be in the normal range before the meal. Information gained from testing foods that contain carbohydrate can 1) help individuals decide whether they need to choose smaller portions of the foods that raise their glucose levels more than others and *2*) help them learn to cover foods with the right amount of diabetes medication.

What is the glycemic load? How can information on glycemic load be used?

The glycemic load (GL) is a calculation of the physiological effects of carbohydrate. It combines the glycemic index (GI) values and the carbohydrate content of an average serving of a food, meal, or day and is defined as the weighted mean of the dietary GI multiplied by the percentage of total energy from carbohydrate. Because the GI is measured for individual foods, an area of discussion has been the ability of the GI to predict glycemic responses to mixed meals (40,41). The GI cannot capture the entire glucose-raising potential of dietary carbohydrates because the blood glucose response is influenced not only by the GI values of a food, but also by the amount of carbohydrate in the food. The concept of GL, therefore, attempts to incorporate both the quality and the quantity of carbohydrate consumed (37).

The GI compared to the GL of a few common foods (based on standard serving sizes) is as follows (42):

Food	Serving Size (carbohydrate g)	GI	GL
Pizza	1 slice (78 g)	86	68
White rice	1 cup (45 g)	102	46
Potatoes	1 (37 g)	102	38
Orange juice	6 oz (20 g)	75	15
White bread	1 slice (13 g)	100	13
Carrots	1/2 cup (8 g)	131	10
Milk	8 oz (11 g)	46	5

This concept has not been tested in clinical studies, but it does seem to combine the two factors that determine glucose response to foods. However, the GL is difficult to use clinically because it cannot be based on equivalent or 15-g carbohydrate servings. It is interesting to note, however, how closely the GL corresponds to the grams of carbohydrate in a serving and not the GI.

There is not enough evidence to suggest exclusive use of either the GI or GL as a method of meal planning for people with diabetes. Instead, place the initial focus on the total amount of carbohydrate eaten. The GL and GI can be used to help patients understand why carbohydrate counting alone may not always be perfect.

First consideration is given to the total amount of carbohydrate when evaluating the glycemic response to a meal. However, there are other variables that can also influence postprandial responses, such as the premeal glucose level, large amounts of fiber or fat, and the GL of the meal.

What are the advantages and disadvantages of so-called "sugar-free" foods that use one or more polyols (sugar alcohols) and/or no-calorie sweeteners (sugar substitutes) as a sweetening ingredient for people with diabetes?

Polyols, also referred to as sugar alcohols, are a group of low-digestible carbohydrates that provide a range of 0.2–3.0 kcal/g (43). These are considered by the Food and Drug Administration (FDA) to be GRAS substances— Generally Recognized as Safe. Their primary use by food manufacturers is to replace either sugars and/or fat to produce foods lower in calories, sugar, and/or fat. Common foods sweetened with polyols are gum, sugar-free candy and cookies, and ice cream. The advantage of foods sweetened with polyols is that they may contain fewer calories than the regularly sweetened food, although, the difference in calories is generally small. This is due to the fact that polyols are only partially absorbed from the small intestine and, therefore, may produce a lower blood glucose excursion than fructose, sucrose, or glucose (2). For this reason, FDA allows manufacturers of products that contain polyols to count the grams of carbohydrate as 2 kcal/g or as the exact calories provided per gram, rather than 4 kcal/g. However, no studies indicate that the use of foods with polyols helps people reduce their energy or carbohydrate intake (2). One disadvantage is that excess consumption of polyols can cause a laxative effect and may result in diarrhea, especially in children (2). For this reason, FDA requires manufacturers to put an information statement about potential laxative effects on products whose daily consumption may result in intake in excess of 50 g sorbitol or 20 g mannitol (43).

In the US, there are currently five no-calorie sweeteners approved for use. Other than saccharin, which predated the FDA food additive approval process, acesulfame-K, aspartame, neotame, and sucralose were approved through the FDA's rigorous food additive approval process that determines safety (44). Saccharin, which was linked to cancer for many years, was dropped from the FDA list of cancer-causing chemicals in 2000, and the label of saccharin-containing products no longer requires a health warning (45). All approved no-calorie sweeteners were determined safe for the general public, including people with diabetes and during pregnancy and lactation (1). These no-calorie sweeteners are also approved for use by various worldwide regulatory agencies.

The advantage of no-calorie sweeteners is that they can be used as a sweetening ingredient in foods and beverages without adding calories. No-calorie sweeteners are commonly used in "diet" versions of carbonated and noncarbonated beverages, yogurt, and ice cream and as a table-top sweetener. In the tabletop packets or granular forms, each sweetener contains about 2 calories per sweetness equivalent of a teaspoon of sucrose. Sucrose contributes 16 calories. The 2 calories are from carbohydrate-containing bulking ingredients, such as dextrose or maltodextrins. These no-calorie sweeteners do not cause a rise in glycemia. To date, insufficient data exist to document whether the long-term use of no-calorie sweeteners improves glycemic control or weight loss and maintenance. Substituting foods and beverages with no-calorie sweeteners and substituting a no-calorie sweetener for sugar are two ways to help people decrease their calorie and carbohydrate intake. Encourage people not to replace these calories with other calorie-containing foods. Consider this example: A 12-oz regularly sweetened carbonated beverage contains about 140 calories and 35 g carbohydrate, ~9 tsp sugar. A carbonated beverage sweetened with a no-calorie sweetener contains 0 calories and 0 g carbohydrate.

Today, food manufacturers are creating foods that utilize the assets and diminish the liabilities of both polyols and no-calorie sweeteners. Foods and beverages may contain one or more polyols, a combination of polyols and no-calorie sweeteners, one no-calorie sweetener, or two no-calorie sweeteners. Therefore, it is critical to teach people to be aware of the names of these sweeteners and how to read Nutrition Facts labels and ingredient lists so they can correctly fit these foods into their eating plan.

For people with diabetes, this is an important area for teaching. Many people with diabetes—especially at diagnosis and/or before they receive diabetes self-management training (if ever)—believe that the most important item to eliminate from their food intake is sugar. Their instinct is to reach for foods that have the claim "sugar-free." Many are under the assumption that these foods don't raise blood glucose levels or contain calories. People with diabetes need education in order to make decisions about using these foods properly and integrating them into their eating plan. Review the teaching points in the next question.

If people choose to use foods sweetened with polyols and/or no-calorie sweeteners, how should you teach them to fit these foods into their food plan?

There are several important teaching points to assure that people with diabetes use foods with polyols and no-calorie sweeteners with a full knowledge of their advantages and disadvantages.

Teaching points:

■ Many people with diabetes continue to believe that their primary nutrition goal is to eliminate sugar from their food intake. Therefore, first determine what the person already knows and does. Focus on all sources of carbohydrate intake, rather than simply on sugars.

■ The words "sugar free" on a food label do not necessarily mean calorie free or carbohydrate free. Teach that the "sugar free" claim simply means that the food does not contain one- and two-unit sugars—mono- and disaccharides—e.g., fructose in fruit and lactose in milk.

■ Polyols and no-calorie sweeteners are safe to be consumed by the general public and people with diabetes.

■ Foods with the claim "sugar free" might contain one or more polyols, one or more no-calorie sweeteners, or a combination of polyols and no-calorie sweeteners. The manufacturer needs to identify these ingredients on the ingredient list.

■ Teach the brand and generic names of polyols and no-calorie sweeteners so they may identify them properly on the ingredient list. Some examples are sorbitol, polydextrose, lactitol, and mannitol.

■ Convey that, on average, foods sweetened with polyols may or may not significantly reduce the calorie content of the food compared to the regularly sweetened product or cause a lower rise in their blood glucose. Products sweetened with polyols may also be more costly than the regularly sweetened products.

- People need to know that some foods sweetened with no-calorie sweeteners have practically no calories (e.g., "diet" carbonated beverages), but others contain some calories from other ingredients (e.g., hot cocoa or yogurt).
- Teach how to make wise purchasing decisions. Help them learn to decide how they will fit these foods into their eating plan. These foods should help them achieve their diabetes nutrition goals. It is still important to pay attention to serving sizes and count the grams of carbohydrates if the product contains calories and carbohydrate.
- Encourage people to try a variety of these foods to find ones that they enjoy and that they find are helpful adjuncts to their food choices.
- Provide coupons, samples, recipes, company web sites, or 800 numbers to assist in discovery.
- Teach people how to fit foods with polyols and no-calorie sweeteners into their eating plan, as follows (43):

Total Carbohydrate (g)	Count as
0–5	Do not count
6–10	1/2 carbohydrate serving, 1/2 starch, fruit, or milk or the actual grams of carbohydrate
11–20	1 carbohydrate serving, 1 starch, fruit, or milk or the actual grams of carbohydrate
21–25	1 1/2 carbohydrate servings, 1 1/2 starch, fruit, or milk or the actual grams of carbohydrate
26–35	2 carbohydrate servings, 2 starch, fruit, or milk or the actual grams of carbohydrate

1. If all of the carbohydrate comes from polyols and the grams of carbohydrate are <10 g, consider it a free food.
2. If all the carbohydrate comes from polyols and the grams of polyols are >10 g, then subtract half of the polyol grams from the total carbohydrate and count the remaining grams of carbohydrate into the eating plan.
3. If there are several sources of carbohydrate including polyols, then subtract half of the polyol grams from the total carbohydrate and count the remaining grams of carbohydrate into the eating plan.

Note that in foods sweetened with polyols where the grams of carbohydrate contributed by polyols are calculated at 2 kcal/g, the calorie count might be lower than if the total grams of carbohydrate were calculated at 4 kcal/g. This can be confusing to consumers.

Does a high-fiber diet improve glycemia, lipids, and insulin levels?

Research suggests that large amounts of dietary fiber are necessary to observe benefits on glucose, insulin, or lipids. It is unknown if, in the real world (compared to controlled research settings), people with diabetes can consume enough fiber to see beneficial effects. However, foods containing fiber can have a laxative effect on the digestive tract and contribute to a feeling of satiety. Foods containing fiber should be encouraged, not because of their beneficial effects on glucose, lipids, and insulin, but because of the other contributions they make to a healthy diet.

Fiber is the structural portion of fruits, vegetables, grains, nuts, and legumes. Structural fibers cannot be digested in the human digestive tract and therefore are not absorbed into the bloodstream. Some fibers add bulk to the diet, thus contributing to the feeling of satiety. Other fibers have a laxative effect on the digestive system. Common sources of fiber are wheat, corn, or oat bran; whole grains; legumes (cooked dried peas and beans); nuts; and vegetables and fruits, especially when raw.

Early research on the effects of fiber on glucose and lipids showed great promise. However, many of the studies had methodological errors. For example, studies had several variables such as decreased weight, decreased energy intake, changed proportions of carbohydrate and fat, or changed medication, yet the benefit was ascribed solely to the increased fiber content of the diet. Better-controlled studies report conflicting outcomes. A study in subjects with type 1 diabetes comparing 56 g fiber/day to 16 g/day reported no clinically significant differences on glycemia (46). However, another study in subjects with type 1 diabetes comparing 50 g fiber/day to 15 g/day reported improved glycemic control and a reduction in the number of hypoglycemic events with the high-fiber diet (47). In a well-controlled study in subjects with type 2 diabetes comparing 11 g fiber/1,000 kcal to 27 g fiber/1,000 kcal reported no differences in glucose, insulin, and lipids (48). In contrast, another well-controlled study in subjects with type 2 diabetes comparing 50 g fiber/day to 24 g/day reported improved glycemic control and decreases in insulin and lipid levels from the higher fiber diet (49).

In regard to the cholesterol-lowering effects of dietary fiber, a meta-analysis concluded that various soluble fibers, such as oats or fruits, reduce total and low-density lipoprotein (LDL) cholesterol by similar amounts (50). However, the effect is small within the practical range of intake. For example, 3 g soluble fiber from oats per day (three 1 cup servings of oatmeal equals 9 g of dietary fiber and 3 g of soluble fiber) can decrease total and LDL cholesterol by ~5 mg/dl. The authors concluded that increasing soluble fiber can make only a small contribution to nutrition therapy to lower total and LDL cholesterol.

If a realistic amount of fiber (20 g/day) doesn't help improve blood glucose levels, why should I encourage people to consume more fiber?

A higher fiber intake contributes to health for a variety of reasons, including

- the likelihood of consuming more vitamins, minerals, and other substances for good health (1,2)
- the potential to improve lipids
- regular bowel function and a reduction in the incidence of colon cancer (51)

The Dietary Guidelines for Americans encourage all Americans to consume at least 20–35 g dietary fiber/day (10). However, most Americans consume in the range of 10–13 g. To accomplish the goal of 20–35 g fiber/day, people should consume a variety of fiber-containing food, such as whole grains, fruits, and vegetables (1).

The following are practical tips for people with diabetes to encourage them to consume more dietary fiber.

- Learn where to find dietary fiber on the Nutrition Facts label.
- Understand that an excellent source of fiber has ≥5 g/serving and a good source of fiber has 2.5–4.9 g/serving.
- Choose foods with a high-fiber content, such as whole-grain cereals; grains, such as oats, barley, bulgur, and buckwheat; acorn and butternut squash; cooked and raw greens; dried peas, beans, and lentils; berries; and dried fruit and nuts.
- Look for dry cereals that contain "whole grain." Purchase dry cereals that contain at least 3 g fiber/serving. Consider eating a mixture of several cereals and choose one that contains at least 7 g fiber/serving, such as All Bran with extra fiber, Bran Buds, or Grape-Nuts.
- Choose hot cereals that contain at least 3 g/serving dietary fiber, such as oat bran, oatmeal, or Wheatena.

- Top dry cereal with diced dried fruit, or cook dried fruit into hot cereal.
- Add nuts and/or cut-up dried fruit into yogurt.
- Choose whole-wheat pasta, brown rice, and the whole-grain alternative whenever possible.
- Sprinkle a tablespoon of wheat germ or ground flax seed on dry cereal or cook into hot cereal.
- Look for whole-grain bread that contains 3 g fiber/serving.
- Choose whole-grain crackers that contain at least 2 g fiber/serving.
- Incorporate cooked beans, peas, and lentils into meals; prepare soups, salads, casseroles, and Mexican meals.
- Top salads with leftover grains or cooked beans, peas, or corn.

Patients who use rapid-acting insulin may need to adjust their dose for fiber. The rationale for subtracting the grams of fiber from total carbohydrate is that the mealtime insulin dose should be based on the available carbohydrate content of meals and fiber, not simply on the total carbohydrate. Dietary fiber, a part of the total carbohydrate, should be subtracted because it is not digested and absorbed and, therefore, is not available to raise blood glucose. Teach people that if they eat a food or meal that contains ≥5 g fiber, they should subtract the grams of dietary fiber from the total carbohydrate count. This is an advanced meal-planning concept and may be most helpful for people using insulin-to-carbohydrate ratios. For most people with diabetes, adjusting the fiber content is not necessary.

PROTEIN

How do protein foods affect glucose and insulin levels?

People with diabetes are often advised that 50–60% of the protein they eat will become glucose, and this glucose will enter the bloodstream in 3–4 h. They are also advised that combining protein foods with foods containing carbohydrate will slow the absorption and release of glucose from the carbohydrate foods. However, studies indicate that protein does not affect circulating blood glucose levels. It is the carbohydrate content of a food or meal that determines the peak glucose response after eating, and this response is not influenced by the protein content of the meals although protein is just as potent a stimulant of insulin secretion as carbohydrate.

As early as 1936, Conn and Newburgh (52) reported no effect on blood glucose levels after ingestion of 50 g protein in the form of lean beef. Subjects were fed breakfasts of glucose, carbohydrate, or lean beef. The blood glucose response after the glucose or carbohydrate was as expected. However, there was no increase in blood glucose response after the lean beef even though there was a consistent rise in blood urea nitrogen indicating protein utilization.

More recently, data from Nuttall et al. (53) also indicated that peripheral glucose concentration does not increase after the ingestion of protein foods in subjects with or without diabetes. That study gave subjects with type 2 diabetes 50 g glucose, 50 g protein, or 50 g glucose and 50 g protein combined, then measured the glucose and insulin responses over the next 5 h. The blood glucose response to glucose was as expected, but the glucose response to protein remained stable and then began to decline. When protein and glucose were combined, the peak glucose response was similar to glucose alone. The insulin responses to glucose and protein given separately were similar, but when combined the insulin response was nearly double the response to glucose or protein alone.

Gannon et al. (54) reported on the glucose appearance rate in the general circulation over 8 h following the ingestion of 50 g protein in the form of lean beef or water in subjects with type 2 diabetes. The plasma glucose concentration decreased similarly after both. Plasma insulin levels did not change after water, but after protein, there was a threefold increase in insulin.

Why does the glucose produced from gluconeogenesis of protein in the liver not appear in the general circulation? The answer is unknown at this time. It has been speculated that the insulin stimulated by dietary protein causes the glucose formed to be rapidly stored as glycogen in the liver and/or in skeletal muscle. The glucose can then be released when insulin levels are low or glucagon levels are elevated, and the original source of the glucose—carbohydrate or protein—cannot be identified.

Therefore, in people with controlled diabetes, minimal, if any, amounts of hepatic glucose are released into the general circulation after the ingestion of foods containing protein. Although protein ingestion increases insulin release in all people, in obese people with type 2 diabetes, the insulin release is greater than in subjects who do not have diabetes (53,55).

Furthermore, as noted in the Nuttall study and numerous other studies (56), combining protein with foods containing carbohydrate does not delay the peak glucose response compared to the ingestion of foods containing carbohydrate alone.

Do people with diabetes require more protein than people without diabetes?

Protein requirements in people with diabetes are related to degree of glycemic control. It had been assumed that in people with diabetes, availability of insulin had minimal effects on protein metabolism and therefore on protein requirements, especially compared to insulin requirements and glucose. However, a number of studies have refuted this view. Moderate hyperglycemia can contribute to an increased turnover of protein in people with diabetes (57,58). Because of the "cost" of this more rapid turnover of protein, the maintenance of body composition, such as lean body mass, and nitrogen requires sufficient energy and protein intakes. Nitrogen equilibrium is not supported with insufficient protein intake.

In people with type 2 diabetes, to obtain positive nitrogen balance requires glycemic control and adequate protein intakes, especially when energy intake is restricted, to maintain lean body mass while selectively mobilizing fat (59). Fortunately, the large amount of protein in the customary diet of people with diabetes compensates for the increased protein catabolism and protects them from protein malnutrition.

In people with type 1 diabetes, insulin deficiency increases protein breakdown with oxidation of essential amino acids (60). Gluconeogenesis is also increased and hepatic extraction of alanine, a key amino acid gluconeogenic precursor, is accelerated. Excessive rate of hepatic glucose production, proteolysis, and amino acid oxidation are all reduced by adequate insulin administration. Therefore, normalization of protein metabolism requires long-term metabolic control and not additional intake of protein. Today, with improved glycemic management in type 1 diabetes, normal protein synthesis, breakdown, and oxidation should occur.

Does eating high-protein foods increase risk for renal disease?

Despite the widespread belief that protein ingestion can influence the development of renal disease, dietary intake of protein is reported to be similar in people with or without nephropathy. In general, average protein intake is ~16–17% of energy intake (~1.4–1.6g/kg/day) and rarely exceeds 20% of calories (56).

However, protein intakes >20% of energy intake may be of concern. In a cross-sectional, clinic-based study (EURODIAB IDDM Complications Study) of >2,500 indi-

viduals with type 1 diabetes, in those whom protein intake
was >20% of energy intake (22% of the patients), average
albumin excretion rates were increased and in the
microalbuminuric range (>20 mg/min) (61). This is in
contrast to people in whom protein intake was <20% of
energy intake who had average albumin excretion rates
(<20 mg/min). In people with macroalbuminuria, 32%
consumed >20% of their energy intake from protein,
whereas this was 23% for the microalbuminuric group
and 20% for the normoalbuminuric group. This was supported by another observational study by Wrone et al.
(62). Protein intake was broken down into quintiles (from
11.7% to >19%). An association between people with diabetes and hypertension in the highest quintile and
microalbuminuria was reported.

Although none of the studies are intervention studies
and thus do not show cause and effect, the EURODIAB
IDDM Complications Study and the Wrone et al. do raise
concern for protein intakes >20% of energy intake. Therefore, it may be prudent for people with diabetes not to
consume protein in excess of 20% of total energy intake
(1). Usual protein intake (<20% of energy) has not shown
a correlation with the development of renal disease.

Is it beneficial to reduce protein intake in the treatment of renal disease?

There is general consensus that controlling blood pressure
with angiotension-converting enzyme inhibitors or angio-
tensin II–receptor blockers, achieving and maintaining
glycemic control, and avoiding smoking are important to
reverse microalbuminuria or slow the rate of decline in
macroalbuminuria. The value of reducing protein intake is
less clear. Accurate evaluation and interpretation of protein studies and nephropathy in diabetes is difficult
because of flaws in study design or choice of outcome
measures, because they were retrospective and uncon-

trolled or not randomized studies, because the stage of nephropathy was unknown, or because they were short-term studies with a small number of patients or poorly documented adherence to the recommended protein intake (63).

Four studies have attempted to reduce protein intake in people with type 1 or type 2 diabetes and microalbuminuria. The achieved protein reductions were on average 1.0 g/kg/day. Even with small reductions in protein intake, the glomerular filtration rate (GFR) improved significantly in all four studies and the albumin excretion rate was reduced significantly in three.

Five studies have been conducted in subjects with type 1 diabetes and macroalbuminuria (i.e., overt nephropathy). The achieved protein reductions were on average 0.8 g/kg/day. Reduced protein intake slowed the decline in the GFR significantly over 33–35 months (64,65). However, a recent study compared a low-protein eating plan (0.6 g/kg/day) with an eating plan free of restrictions (66). Hypertension and glycemia had been under control for at least 3 months before beginning the study. Not only were the average decline in GFR comparable in both groups, of concern was a decrease in values of serum pre-albumin and serum albumin observed in the low-protein group, revealing that severe protein restriction may cause malnutrition.

The 2002 American Diabetes Association nutrition guidelines state that there is evidence for reducing protein intake with microalbuminuria. Reducing protein intake to 0.8–1.0 g/kg/day is associated with renal improvement. (Note that this level of protein is consistent with the current Recommended Daily Allowance for healthy adults and should not be considered low protein.) With the onset of clinical nephropathy, evidence shows that lowering protein intake to ≤0.8 g/kg/day may slow progression toward end-stage renal disease. Protein status should be monitored closely so that the person's nutritional status is not compromised.

The differing effects of animal and vegetable protein on renal function has been controversial. In a study comparing animal versus plant protein meals in people with type 2 diabetes and microalbuminuria, both diets improved renal function, lipids, glycemia, and blood pressure (67). Following a weight-maintaining, healthy plan of eating, regardless of the protein source, appears to be beneficial.

What are nutrition and physical activity recommendations for metabolic syndrome?

The metabolic syndrome is a cluster of factors such as dyslipidemia, hypertension, intra-abdominal obesity, and glucose intolerance that are associated with insulin resistance. Therefore, the question becomes, what nutrition and physical activity recommendations affect insulin resistance? Although the effect of the composition of the eating plan (e.g., percentage of carbohydrate and fats) on insulin resistance is debatable (see below), increased physical activity and decreased energy intake are the keys to reducing insulin resistance (68). Both the increase in physical activity and the decrease in energy intake increase insulin sensitivity, with or without weight loss.

It is often assumed that foods containing carbohydrate affect insulin resistance because they stimulate insulin release, and therefore, foods containing carbohydrate should be restricted. However, research suggests that carbohydrate improves insulin sensitivity (69). It also has been suggested that sucrose and fructose, in particular, increase insulin resistance. Studies in rats demonstrated that high sucrose (>60% of energy intake) or fructose (>34% of energy intake) intake causes a decline in insulin sensitivity, which is a function of the dose and duration of exposure. However, studies in humans using more usual amounts of sucrose or fructose have shown no effect on insulin sensitivity from either (70).

Carbohydrate and fat intake tend to go hand in hand. When carbohydrate intake increases, fat intake decreases, and when carbohydrate intake decreases, fat intake increases. Protein intake tends to remain remarkably consistent. Therefore, the improvement in insulin sensitivity with an increase in carbohydrate may be because of the lowering of fat intake. There are numerous observational studies linking high fat intake, regardless of the type of fat (except for omega-3), with insulin resistance (71). On the other hand, some intervention studies with monounsaturated fats (or polyunsaturated fats) report improvements in insulin sensitivity (72). Saturated fats are associated with insulin resistance, so they clearly should be decreased to improve insulin sensitivity.

Walking for as little as 150–160 min/week is enough to lower insulin resistance. Physical activity increases the affinity of the insulin receptor for insulin, the mobilization of glucose transporters, and the activity of tyrosine kinase, each of which leads to decreased insulin resistance in skeletal muscle (73). Similarly, as little as a 5% decrease in body weight results in improvements in insulin resistance. However, long-term studies on weight loss and insulin sensitivity are not available. The best advice for improving insulin resistance continues to be to eat less and be more active.

FAT

What are the differences between the nutrition recommendations of the American Diabetes Association (ADA), the American Heart Association (AHA), and the National Cholesterol Education Program (NCEP) Adult Treatment Panel III (ATP III)? What are the similarities?

Each set of recommendations is intended for a slightly different population. The AHA nutrition guidelines are designed for the general population, with the objective being to decrease the risk of cardiovascular disease by dietary and other lifestyle practices (74). A major strength of the AHA recommendations is that they provide food selection guidelines that are easily interpreted by the general public.

The NCEP ATP III updates clinical guidelines for cholesterol testing and clinical management of elevated cholesterol (75). Although ATP III's attention is to intensive treatment of patients with coronary artery disease, including therapeutic lifestyle changes, a major new feature of ATP III is attention to primary prevention in people with multiple risk factors. A major strength of the NCEP guidelines is that nutrition therapy is integrated into the overall management of dyslipidemia, especially therapeutic lifestyle changes for low-density lipoprotein (LDL) cholesterol.

The ADA report provides evidence-based principles and recommendations for nutrition therapy in the treatment and, for the first time, prevention of diabetes (1,2). Because the level of the supporting evidence is clear, nutrition guidelines can be prioritized based on the strength of the evidence. The ADA notes that research supporting their guidelines for cardiovascular disease and lipids is from the general population. Studies in people with diabetes demonstrating the effects of specific percentages of saturated fatty acids (e.g., 10% vs. 7% of energy) on lipid concentrations are not available.

Therefore, although all the organizations review the same research studies, depending on their objectives, they develop nutrition guidelines for their intended populations (76). ADA, AHA, and NCEP all have similar guidelines for the desirable percentages of energy from saturated fat and dietary cholesterol. Foods with a high content of saturated fatty acids should be limited to <10% of total energy intake/day and dietary cholesterol to <300 mg/day. These recommendations help people with diabetes achieve the goal of an LDL cholesterol <100 mg/dl. People who have LDL cholesterol ≥100 mg/dl should limit saturated fatty acids to <7% of total energy intake/day and dietary cholesterol to <200 mg/day.

However, percentage of calories from a nutrient is not very helpful advice for choosing foods because the food label lists grams of fat per serving. It is more helpful to give people a goal in terms of total grams of fat or total grams of saturated fat. For example, the goal is to keep saturated fat to <15 g/day for someone on a lower-calorie diet and to <20 g/day for someone eating ~2,000 calories/day. A helpful tip is to look for foods with 5 g or less of saturated fat/serving.

The three organizations differ slightly in their recommendations for monounsaturated and polyunsaturated fats (see below).

What are the effects of monounsaturated fats and polyunsaturated fats on lipid levels?

Monounsaturated fatty acids (MUFA) and polyunsaturated fatty acids (PUFA) reduce blood cholesterol concentrations when they replace saturated fatty acids in the foods we eat. The American Heart Association notes that in the absence of weight loss, foods high in total carbohydrate (e.g., >55% of energy) can lead to elevated triglycerides and decreased high-density lipoprotein cholesterol. These effects do not occur with substitution of MUFA and PUFA for saturated fat. The National Cholesterol Education Program suggests that MUFA can be up to 20% of total energy and PUFA up to 10% of total energy intake.

The American Diabetes Association is more cautious in recommending increased intake of MUFA or PUFA. Several observational studies report that total dietary fat, regardless of the type of fat, is associated with insulin resistance (71,77). However, other studies in which the food plan was enriched with monounsaturated fats have reported improvements in insulin resistance (78).

Beside the potential of dietary fats to contribute to insulin resistance, another concern is their high energy content. Foods high in MUFA or PUFA selected ad libitum may lead to higher energy intake and weight gain. The major MUFA in foods is oleic, and the major dietary sources of oleic are the same as for saturated fat: dairy, beef, pork, poultry, and lamb. This means that when saturated fat is restricted, so is MUFA. Therefore, to increase MUFA (or PUFA), individuals need to add nuts and oils to the foods they eat. Unless portions sizes are carefully monitored, it may be easy to increase energy intake. Furthermore, to increase MUFA to 20% of energy requires the substitution of oils or nuts (the most common MUFA) for one-fifth of the daily calories, something that is very difficult for many individuals to do.

Therefore, the American Diabetes Association recommends that an individual's metabolic profile and need to lose weight will determine nutrition therapy recommendations. To lower low-density lipoprotein cholesterol, energy from saturated fat can be reduced and not replaced if concurrent weight loss is desirable. If weight loss is not a goal, saturated fats can be replaced with either MUFA or carbohydrate.

Note: The guidelines discussed above are for the *cis* form of MUFA. In natural unsaturated fatty acids, the two carbons participating in a double bond bind a hydrogen on the same side of the bond and thus are the *cis*-isomer form. Hydrogenation of unsaturated fatty acids adds hydrogen to liquid oils to form a solid and stable fat, and in the process, fatty acids are reshaped into *trans* fatty acids. See page 42 for a discussion of *trans* fats.

Does a higher fat intake contribute to a higher caloric intake?

In general, research suggests that low-fat eating plans are usually associated with modest weight loss, which can be maintained as long as the low-fat plan is continued (79). With this modest weight loss, decreases in total cholesterol and triglycerides and an increase in high-density lipoprotein cholesterol are observed.

Conversely, eating plans high in fat also tend to be higher in energy intake (80,81,33). Thus far, all published research regarding the substitution of monounsaturated fatty acids for saturated fat or carbohydrate has been done in controlled settings where food is provided. This is done to determine accurately what people are eating. What happens when free-living people ad libitum substitute monounsaturated fatty acids (or polyunsaturated fatty acids) for saturated fat or carbohydrate is unknown. Generally, as fat intake increases so does the energy content of the total food intake. Research supports the statement that reduced-fat meal plans maintained over the long-term contribute to weight loss and improvements in dyslipidemia.

What advice can I give to individuals to help them reduce their fat intake and/or to eat more healthy fats?

The bottom line is that individuals must pay attention to the total amount of saturated fat and calories they eat. There is no "magic bullet." The following are some tips that can help person with diabetes lower their intake of saturated fat (82).

- Eat smaller and fewer meat servings. Most adults should limit total meat intake to about 6 oz after cooking/day. Some women need only 4–5 oz/day. People on meal plans of >2,000 calories may be able to have up to 8 oz meat/day.
- Choose leaner cuts of meats such as beef and pork tenderloin, fish, or poultry (without skin). Look for luncheon meats with 3 g or less of fat/oz.
- Choose high-fat meat servings no more than two or three times a week. Regular luncheon meats, other processed meats, frankfurters, sausage, bacon, and prime cuts of meat are high-fat meats.
- Cook using low-fat cooking methods such as baking, broiling, or roasting. When frying or sautéing foods,

use nonfat cooking spray or a small amount of vegetable oil.

- Chill gravies, soups, or stews until the fat hardens. Remove the fat layer, reheat, and serve.
- Drink fat-free or 1% milk.
- Use plain nonfat yogurt (2 Tbsp contain <20 calories) instead of sour cream (2 Tbsp contain 50 calories) or mayonnaise (2 Tbsp contain 200 calories) as a condiment or in recipes for dips and salad dressings.
- Also, try some of the many light or low-fat sour creams, mayonnaise, and salad dressings on the market. Using fat replacers, which have 1–2 kcal/g fat compared to 9 kcal/g fat, helps lower total fat intake.
- Choose cheeses that have 5 g or less of fat/oz.
- Use a soft margarine or one made with a plant stanol or sterol ester instead of butter, but be careful of amounts. The calories in margarine and butter are the same, but because butter is primarily a saturated fat, margarine is recommended. Look for margarine that lists a liquid oil such as corn, safflower, or soybean oil as the first ingredient. A soft or tub margarine is a better choice than solid or stick margarine. Better yet, look for a light (lower-fat and -calorie) tub margarine.
- Use a healthier liquid oil, such as canola or olive oil, to do all sautéing and cooking rather than margarine, butter, or shortening.
- Choose low-fat or fat-free salad dressings. One tablespoon of a low-fat or fat-free salad dressing generally has <20 calories and is considered a "free food;" two or three tablespoons is one fat serving. One tablespoon of a regular dressing is one fat serving, which is ~5 g fat and 45 calories. Limit fat servings to one per meal.
- Many fat-free products such as salad dressings and sour cream contain carbohydrate. Check the nutrition label to determine if your serving size should be counted as a carbohydrate serving.

What are the advantages and disadvantages of lower-fat and fat-free foods for people with diabetes?

Manufacturers of lower-fat and fat-free foods can create foods with reduced calories and improved fat qualities with the use of a group of ingredients referred to as fat replacers. Fat replacers mimic various properties of fat. Today, fat replacers are most often carbohydrate-based ingredients, such as modified food starch, polydextrose, and guar gum. In addition, some available fat replacers are protein or fat based. Most fat replacers are approved by Food and Drug Administration as GRAS substances— Generally Recognized as Safe (44).

Encourage people with diabetes, who also often have abnormal lipid levels, to decrease their intake of saturated fat and cholesterol (1). Lower-fat and fat-free foods that contain fat replacers may help people achieve their lipid goals as well as reduce total energy intake (83). The disadvantages of these products are that the calorie savings may not be large enough to make an impact on helping the person achieve their nutrition goals and the taste of some products may be less than desirable. In addition, because many of the currently used fat replacers are carbohydrate based, these foods may be lower in fat content but higher in carbohydrate content with minimal caloric savings.

Encourage people to try a variety of these products and find ones that they enjoy and help them achieve their nutrition goals. They should be encouraged to try lower-fat or fat-free milk, margarines, spread, cream cheese, sour cream, mayonnaise, salad dressing, and snack foods.

Teaching points:

- Provide an understanding of the category of ingredients called fat replacers and their common names in ingredient lists. Examples of names are modified food starch, guar gum, xanthin, and maltodextrins.
- Teach the meaning of the nutrition claims used on these products, such as fat free, reduced fat, low fat, and less fat.

- Teach that the terms low fat, reduced fat, and fat free don't necessarily mean calorie or carbohydrate free. Teach that the carbohydrate content of these foods may be higher with a minimal calorie savings.
- Show people food labels with the Nutrition Facts and ingredient lists from regular and lower-fat products to demonstrate the calorie and fat comparisons of both maximally and minimally helpful products. For example, fat-free milk and light sour cream would provide significant calorie and fat reductions compared to whole milk and regular sour cream. But fat-free or low-fat crackers compared to regular crackers may only represent a minimal calorie or fat savings.

Should I recommend one of the margarine-like spreads that contain plant stanol esters (Benecol) or plant sterol esters (Take Control)?

Products on the market such as Benecol and Take Control are spreads fortified with plant stanol or sterol esters. These esters are derived from either wood or soybean oil and are effective in providing an additional low-density lipoprotein (LDL) cholesterol–lowering benefit when added to diets that are already low in saturated fat and cholesterol (84). Plant stanol and sterol esters block the intestinal absorption of dietary and biliary cholesterol. Research shows that ingestion of ~2 g/day of plant stanol/sterol esters decreases total and LDL cholesterol by ~10% (2,11). In a multicenter, double-blind, and placebo-controlled trial of hypercholesterolemic patients, the spread containing plant sterol ester reduced LDL cholesterol from baseline by 17% (85). The nutrition recommendations of both the American Diabetes Association and the National Cholesterol Education Program Adult Treatment Panel III mention the therapeutic option of using plant stanols/sterol esters (~2 g/day) to lower LDL cholesterol (1,11).

In 2002, the Food and Drug Administration published a Health Claim Final Rule for plant sterol/stanol esters. The new rule permits manufacturers to state on package labels and in advertising that consuming the appropriate number of servings of foods containing plant sterol esters or plant stanol esters will reduce the risk of heart disease. To make this claim, the food product must also be low in saturated fat, low in cholesterol, and contain 0.65 g plant sterol esters or 1.7 g plant stanol esters per reference amount commonly consumed (85).

These spreads may help lower elevated cholesterol levels, particularly LDL cholesterol levels in people with diabetes. In addition, they may be a helpful adjunct to decreasing total fat, particularly saturated fat, from food sources. These products are more expensive than other spreads. Other lifestyle modifications that can lower LDL cholesterol levels include decreasing total fat and saturated fat, increasing monounsaturated fat and physical activity, and losing modest amounts of weight. These spreads offer a useful adjunct to other lifestyle changes known to improve lipid levels.

What is the benefit of increasing omega-3 fatty acid intake? How much is recommended? Are supplements like fish oil or omega-3 capsules better than eating foods that contain omega-3 fatty acids? What about the concerns regarding the mercury content of fish?

Studies show that omega-3 polyunsaturated fatty acids lower plasma triglyceride levels in people with type 2 diabetes (2). They are probably the most beneficial in people with severe hypertriglyceridemia and positively affect platelet aggregation and thrombogenecity (11). Most studies using omega-3 fatty acids in foods have been conducted in the general population, so limited data are available in people with diabetes. However, there appears to be a cardioprotective effect from omega-3 fatty acids in foods.

In a recent study investigating fish and omega-3 fatty acid intake on the risk of heart disease in women with diabetes, a higher consumption of fish and long-chain omega-3 fatty acids was associated with a lower coronary heart disease incidence (86). In this study, they calculated a 6- to 8-oz portion of fish to have ~1.16 g long-chain omega-3 fatty acids (86).

The American Diabetes Association recommends consuming 2–3 servings of fish/week and/or other foods that contain omega-3 fatty acids (1). Good omega-3 fatty acid (eicosapentaenoic acid and docosahexaenoic acid) sources of food include nonpredator, fatty, dark-meat fish such as salmon, mackerel, sardines, and herring and plant sources such as flaxseed, soybeans, and walnuts.

People with severe triglyceridemia may benefit from a supplement (fish oil or omega-3 capsules) of 2–4 g omega-3 fatty acid/day. Even the 1-g/day dose (~6–8 oz of the recommended types of fish) recommended by the American Heart Association for people with cardiovascular disease may be more than many people can get from eating food alone (11). Concerns have been raised that fish oil may worsen glycemic control by diverting substrates from lipogenesis to gluconeogenesis in the process of inhibiting hepatic triglyceride synthesis (87). Two recent meta-analyses, however, found no significant adverse effects of fish oil supplementation on glycemic control, and the fish oil supplementation lowered triglyceride levels by ~30% (88,89).

Some types of fish may contain significant levels of mercury, PCBs, dioxins, and other environmental contaminants. Levels of these substances are generally highest in older and larger predatory fish and marine mammals. Eating a variety of fish will help minimize any potentially adverse effects due to environmental pollutants (11).

What are *trans* fats, and should people with diabetes lower their *trans* fat intake?

Trans fats are created through the process of hydrogenation that solidifies liquid oils. *Trans* fats are found in many foods such as vegetable shortenings, margarines, potato chips, crackers, cookies, cakes, pies, doughnuts, and convenience and restaurant foods that are fried, such as chicken, fish, and potatoes. Most *trans* fats in foods come from processed foods, whereas only about one-fifth of *trans* fats come from unprocessed animal sources, such as meat and dairy products. The purpose of hydrogenation, according to the Food and Drug Administration, is that it helps manufacturers increase the shelf life and flavor stability of vegetable oils. In the American diet, *trans* fats provide only ~3% of total energy intake compared to ~11% from saturated fat and 34% from total fat (76).

Studies indicate that consumption of *trans* fats contributes to increased low-density lipoprotein cholesterol and decreased high-density lipoprotein cholesterol levels, which increase the risk for heart disease. In a longitudinal and comprehensive clinical study about dietary fat and the risk of type 2 diabetes reported in 2001, results indicated a 1.39 relative risk of developing type 2 diabetes with a 2% increase in energy from *trans* fats (11). Total fat intake, compared with equivalent energy intake from carbohydrate, was not associated with risk of type 2 diabetes. Intakes of saturated and monounsaturated fats were also not significantly associated with type 2 diabetes.

People can lower their intake of *trans* fat in several ways. First, decrease total fat intake, especially from commercial foods such as margarine, cookies, crackers, frozen convenience foods, and restaurant foods that have been deep-fat fried. Instead, purchase a margarine that is low in *trans* fat, such as a liquid or tub margarine. When using oil, choose the healthier monounsaturated fats such as olive or canola oil.

Finally, decrease saturated fat intake. Saturated fats represent the highest percentage of our total fat intake, ~13%. Because *trans* fats are added to food, it may be easier to cut back, eliminate, or find a substitute for these foods. Saturated fats are found naturally in foods such as meats and dairy products, and it may be more difficult to reduce their intake. A good start, however, would be to eat the leanest cuts of meats or eat meat less often and to eat/drink low-fat or fat-free dairy products.

ALCOHOL

What are the recommendations for alcohol intake in people with diabetes? What effect does alcohol ingestion have on glucose and insulin levels?

Alcohol recommendations for adults with diabetes are similar to those for the general public. Alcoholic drinks should be limited to two or less per day for men and one or less per day for women. Less alcohol is recommended for women because after consuming comparable amounts of alcohol, women have higher blood ethanol concentrations than men, even with allowances for size differences. Women, compared to men, have an increased bioavailability of alcohol resulting from decreased gastric first-phase metabolism and decreased gastric alcohol dehydrogenase activity, which may contribute to the enhanced susceptibility of women to the effects of alcohol (90).

One drink is defined as a 12 oz beer, 5 oz wine, or 1.5 oz distilled sprits, each of which contains ~15 g alcohol. Alcoholic beverages are considered an addition to the regular meal plan. No food should be omitted. Regular beer, because it generally contains ~15 g carbohydrate, can be counted as one carbohydrate serving (which equals 15 g carbohydrate). If amounts are limited to the recommended amounts, sweet wines or light beer do not need to be counted as carbohydrate servings.

The effect of alcoholic beverages depends on how much an individual drinks, whether alcohol use is chronic and excessive, whether alcohol is consumed with or without food, and whether an individual is on insulin or an insulin secretegogue. Research in people with type 1 or type 2 diabetes who acutely drank moderate amounts of alcohol (about three drinks or <45 g alcohol) with food showed no effect from alcohol on blood glucose or insulin levels (91). In contrast, chronic ingestion (≥45 g/day) can cause deterioration in both short- and long-term blood glucose control. However, the effects from excessive alcohol are reversed after abstinence for 3 days (92).

For individuals using insulin or insulin secretegogues, alcohol should be consumed with food to prevent hypoglycemia. Alcohol without food can lower blood glucose levels because alcohol is not metabolized into glucose. Therefore, if individuals drink without eating, there is no immediate source of glucose available, and hypoglycemia can result. Evening consumption of alcohol can also increase the risk of hypoglycemia the next morning (93). This is associated with reduced nocturnal growth hormone secretion. Blood glucose checking can be used to determine whether extra carbohydrate or a reduction in the morning insulin dose is needed.

The type of alcoholic beverage ingested does not make a difference. All alcoholic beverages begin as carbohydrates (e.g., grains or fruits) and are converted to alcohol during the process of fermentation. Distillation continues this process, and the percentage of alcohol in distilled beverages is the percentage of conversion of carbohydrate distilled into alcohol. The same precautions that apply to the general population regarding the use of alcohol also apply to people with diabetes. People who should not drink include women during pregnancy and people with medical problems such as pancreatitis, advanced neuropathy, or alcohol abuse.

Are there health benefits from moderate intake of alcoholic beverages?

Epidemiological studies suggest a U- or J-shaped benefit from moderate consumption of alcohol (~15–30 g/day). For example, in nondiabetic adults, light-to-moderate amounts of alcohol are associated with a decreased risk of type 2 diabetes (94,95), coronary heart disease (96,97), stroke (98), and increased insulin sensitivity (99,100).

In adults with type 2 diabetes, light-to-moderate amounts of alcohol (5–15 g/day) are associated with a decreased risk of coronary heart disease, perhaps due to the reported ability of alcohol to increase high-density lipoprotein cholesterol (99,100). It should be noted that benefits are reported from observational studies and, therefore, should be taken with caution. Remember the reported benefits of antioxidant vitamins from observational and short-term intervention studies? When large intervention clinical trials were conducted, the results from earlier studies were not replicated. Prospective long-term studies are needed to confirm observations.

Adults with diabetes can consider drinking small amounts of alcohol, because alcohol raises high-density lipoprotein cholesterol levels. However, if individuals don't drink now, they shouldn't start. Regular exercise can have the same potential benefit as moderate amounts of alcohol and for many people will be more appropriate.

What is the effect of alcohol on blood pressure and triglycerides?

Although it is often assumed that alcohol raises both blood pressure and triglycerides, the effect depends on the amount of alcohol ingested. For instance, light-to-moderate amounts of alcohol do not raise blood pressure; however, excessive amounts (>30–60 g/day) can elevate blood pressure levels (101,102). This again illustrates the importance of light-to-moderate alcohol consumption.

The effect of alcohol on triglycerides is similar. Excessive amounts of alcohol increase VLDL synthesis (103), an effect that is enhanced by genetics, a high-fat diet, and diabetes. However, two drinks per day in subjects with fasting hypertriglyceridemia did not increase triglycerides (104). Also, ingestion of 30 g/day of alcohol beneficially affected triglyceride levels and improved insulin sensitivity in nondiabetic women (100). These studies suggest that even adults with hypertriglyceridemia may occasionally drink alcohol in moderation.

The message is always the same. Avoid large intakes of alcoholic beverages for the described reasons. But if a person chooses to occasionally have a "drink," they can do so knowing they are likely not causing adverse health effects and may actually be gaining some health benefits.

What are the most important concepts to teach people with type 1 and type 2 diabetes about alcohol consumption?

Alcohol has the potential to cause hypoglycemia and hyperglycemia (105). Different reactions to alcohol intake are observed based on the person's current blood glucose level, medication action curve(s), and whether they are fasting. The hypoglycemia that can be caused by alcohol intake in people taking insulin secretegogues can be worse than hypoglycemia caused for other reasons.

According to the American Diabetes Association nutrition recommendations (1), blood glucose levels will not be affected by the moderate use of alcohol when circumstances are normal and diabetes is well controlled. Moderate use of alcohol is defined in these recommendations and in the United States Department of Agriculture Dietary Guidelines (10) as no more than two drinks per day for men and no more than one drink per day for women.

Definition of one drink:

- 12 oz beer
- 5 oz wine (any type)
- 1.5 oz distilled spirits (i.e., hard liquor)

The following people should abstain from alcohol consumption:

- pregnant women
- women attempting to get pregnant
- people with frequent hypoglycemia and/or hypoglycemia unawareness
- people with severely elevated triglycerides
- people with pancreatitis
- people with advanced neuropathy

Teaching points:

- People with type 1 diabetes may have a risk of late onset hypoglycemia with alcohol intake. For this reason, people with type 1 diabetes should consume alcohol along with food. They should also be taught about the risk of and treatment for hypoglycemia.
- People with type 1 diabetes should not omit food from their eating plan to substitute for the calories of alcohol. This may exacerbate the risk of hypoglycemia (1).
- The risk of alcohol-induced hypoglycemia in people with type 2 diabetes, especially those not taking an insulin secretegogue, is minimal.
- People with type 2 diabetes rarely have sufficient grams of fat allotted in their eating plan to have a surplus to omit fat for alcohol intake. The most realistic advice is to consume a minimal amount of alcohol in addition to regular food intake but to caution about the extra calories of alcohol (1).
- Drink safely and smartly. Follow all precautions that are encouraged for the general population (e.g., drink in moderation, don't drink and drive).
- Drink alcohol only if glycemic levels are within target ranges.

- If a person has consumed alcohol and will be driving, check blood glucose before doing so. If blood glucose is low, eat something before driving and/or designate someone else to drive.
- Know blood glucose level before consuming alcohol. If blood glucose is low, eat something to raise it.
- If alcohol is consumed in the evening and/or at night and the person uses a diabetes medication that can cause hypoglycemia, monitor blood glucose before going to sleep. If it is near low or low, eat something to raise it. Hypoglycemia can occur several hours after consuming alcohol.
- Hypoglycemia and drunkenness have some similar symptoms. At times, people with diabetes and hypo-glycemia have been mistaken for being drunk and did not receive the proper treatment to resolve the hypo-glycemia. This is a good reason to suggest wearing dia-betes identification.
- Before prescribing metformin, clinicians should assess the person's drinking habits. Regular binge drinking while taking metformin could increase the risk of lactic acidosis.
- To decrease the amount of alcoholic drinks consumed in social situations, also drink noncaloric and nonalco-holic beverages, such as water, club soda, diet tonic water, iced tea, and diet soda.

SUPPLEMENTS

How should I find out whether people are taking vitamin and mineral supplements? What should I do if they are taking supplements that are contraindicated for them or if they are taking unsafe doses?

1. Always ask what supplements they are taking, how much, how often, and why.

- Ask gently and reserve comment. People often don't share information about alternative therapies. This question can also be included on a nutrition assessment form—patients may be more willing to disclose their habits in writing rather than in a face-to-face interview.
- Many people do not remember what supplements they are taking. Request they bring in a printed list or the containers.
- The person may be getting the same supplement from multiple sources.
- Compare vitamin and mineral totals with a Daily Reference Intake or the Tolerable Upper Intake Level.
- Assess their total food intake. Are there nutrients missing in their usual intake? For example, if they do not drink milk, they may get inadequate calcium unless they take a supplement.

2. What medications do they take?

- Some supplements interact or compound the action of a prescription drug or over-the-counter medications. For example, coumadin, ginkgo biloba, aspirin, dong quai, vanadium, and vitamin E all have anticoagulant properties. St. John's Wort may reduce the effectiveness of prescription drugs for heart disease, depression, and contraception (106).
- Note drug/disease interaction. Conditions/medical problems such as gastrointestinal, renal, and blood pressure disorders affect absorption.
- Ask about medical nutritional supplements (which can include drinks, herbs, and bars in addition to vitamin and mineral tablets), many of which contain 25–50% of the Daily Reference Intake for some vitamins or minerals.
- St. John's Wort changes the action of digoxin, warfarin, antidepressants, and oral contraceptives.

3. Do not assume that if a supplement doesn't help, at least it won't hurt.

- Natural does not mean healthy and/or safe (e.g., poisonous mushrooms are natural).
- The absence of label warnings does not imply safety. The manufacturer decides what to include on the label.

4. Evaluate the source of the patient's information in support of taking vitamin and mineral supplements.

- Is it published by the government, a university, or a reputable medical or health organization?
- Has it been reviewed by experts?
- Does it document sources or make general statements?
- Is the information current?
- Does it sound too good to be true?
- Was the conclusion drawn from a single study or body of research?
- Is it consistent with other information you have read?

Report adverse events directly to Food and Drug Administration whenever you think a product caused a serious problem.

- 1-800-FDA-1088
- 1-800-FDA-0178
- www.fda.gov/medwatch/how.htm

For more information and to stay abreast of changes, refer to the US Food and Drug Administration Center for Food Safety and Applied Nutrition Dietary Supplements at http://www.cfsan.fda.gov/~dms/supplmnt.html

Are antioxidant supplements, such as vitamin E, of benefit to people with diabetes?

The Institute of Medicine of the National Academies in Washington, DC, assembles authorities in nutrition and medicine to determine nutrient Dietary Reference Intakes for health and disease. After reviewing all the evidence,

they concluded that megadoses of antioxidants—
vitamin C, vitamin E, selenium, beta-carotene, and
other carotenoids—have not been proven to protect
against heart and vessel diseases, diabetes, or various
forms of cancer (107). In fact, they concluded that the
opposite may be true: high doses of antioxidants may
lead to health problems, including diarrhea, bleeding,
and toxic reactions.

The potential role of antioxidant supplements to prevent the oxidative modification of lipoproteins was based
on a large number of observational epidemiological studies and a small number of intervention studies with a limited number of subjects and of relatively short duration.
However, large randomized trials in which antioxidants
were compared to placebos have contradicted the claims
that antioxidant vitamins have a role in preventing cardiovascular disease in the general public and in people with
diabetes, and in some instances, evidence as to potential
adverse outcomes from antioxidant vitamins has emerged
(108). For example, a meta-analysis assessed the effects of
alpha-tocopherol (vitamin E) and beta-carotene on long-
term cardiovascular mortality and morbidity (109). Seven
randomized trials of vitamin E treatment and eight of
beta-carotene treatment were analyzed, and all included
1,000 or more patients. Doses of vitamin E ranged from
50–800 IU and doses of beta-carotene from 15–50 mg.
Follow-up occurred from 1.4 to 12 years. The vitamin E
trials involved a total of 81,788 patients and vitamin E did
not provide benefit in mortality compared with controls
or significantly decrease the risk of cardiovascular death.
The beta-carotene trials involved over 138,113 patients
and beta-carotene led to a small but significant increase in
all-cause mortality and a slight increase in cardiovascular
death.

In addition, two studies with beta-carotene found an
unexplained increase in lung cancer in people taking beta-
carotene (110,111). In regard to vitamin E, of interest is

the Heart Outcomes Prevention Evaluation trial, which included 9,541 people, 39% of whom had diabetes (112). Supplementation with 400 IU/day vitamin E for 4.5 years failed to show any benefit from the supplement. Of concern are recent clinical trials reporting that antioxidants may hamper the beneficial effects of simvastatin and niacin on lipid profile, specifically high-density lipoprotein cholesterol (113,114).

Therefore, the American Diabetes Association nutrition technical review concluded that routine supplementation of the diet with antioxidants is not advised because of the uncertainties relating to long-term benefit and safety (2). Instead, emphasize established interventions—lifestyle strategies, aspirin, lipid- and hypertension-lowering medications, and smoking cessation—to lower risk of cardiovascular disease.

SODIUM

Does everyone with diabetes need to restrict their sodium intake?

Everyone with diabetes may benefit from limiting sodium, but after assessing the situation, you may or may not decide that lowering sodium intake is a priority at this time. Because typical sodium intake is well beyond the minimum requirement, it is unlikely that eating less salt/sodium would be a medical problem and may be a helpful habit to develop, as age increases the likelihood of hypertension or fluid retention.

For people with hypertension, reducing sodium intake from 4,600 mg/day to 2,300 mg/day lowered blood pressure 5 mmHg diastolic and 2–3 mmHg systolic (19). There are no studies to document the same effect in people with diabetes, but by expert consensus, the recommendation for people with diabetes and hypertension is to limit sodium to ≤2,400 mg/day (115) An estimated 20–60% of the people with diabetes also have hypertension (1). Not all of these individuals are "sodium sensitive" (19). However, because there is no way to assess that trait and because sodium restriction enhances the benefit of hypertensive medications, limiting sodium or at least avoiding excesses of sodium intake would seem prudent for all people with diabetes and mild-to-moderate hypertension.

For those without hypertension, the recommended sodium intake is the same as for the general population: 2,400–3,000 mg/day. For those with severe hypertension, edema, or nephropathy, sodium intake <2,000 mg/day is advised.

Other considerations:

1. Is hypertension (or fluid retention) the priority clinical issue right now? Or is an elevated glycated hemoglobin A1C, frequent hypoglycemia, or a nonhealing ulcer a more pressing concern?
2. Does the person know how to limit sodium? Depending on patient's current habits, some ideas are:

- Remove the salt shaker from the table.
- Cook with less salt. Try herbs, spices, lemon juice, garlic, and onion to flavor food.
- Limit high-sodium foods like dill pickles, sauerkraut, potato/corn chips, processed meats, canned soups, and sauces like ketchup, soy sauce, and steak sauce.
- Eat unprocessed food prepared at home more often than processed and restaurant foods.
- When eating out, choose plain foods (e.g., grilled chicken and baked potato) rather than combination foods (e.g., chicken potpie). Limit fast foods, which tend to be higher in sodium than foods at sit-down restaurants.
- Use fresh or frozen instead of canned vegetables.

- Choose fresh meat (e.g., pork loin) instead of cured meat (e.g., ham).
- Try Healthy Choice soups or frozen entrees. This brand is consistently modified for sodium as well as sugar and fat.
- Include fruit. There is very little sodium in fresh or canned fruit.

3. Would an alternate approach to the same goal be more effective? If hypertension is the reason to limit sodium, weight loss, exercise, or moderation of alcohol intake may do the same. The Dietary Approaches to Stop Hypertension diet, a combination of increased fruits and vegetables with low-fat dairy, has also been shown to improve hypertension (20), and in some people, weight loss is as effective as a first-line hypertensive medication (21).

Nutrition Assessment

How can I assess the readiness of an overweight person to make changes in their lifestyle to improve their diabetes control?

People who are not ready or are unwilling to lose weight rarely succeed in a weight loss program (116). Once a person at increased medical risk for premature death or illness from overweight or obesity has been identified, the medical history and physical examination should include potential causes and complications of obesity, and the person's readiness to lose weight should be determined.

The following issues help the health care provider evaluate a person's readiness to make lifestyle changes necessary to achieve and maintain a lower weight (117,118):

- reasons for wanting to lose weight
- support the person expects from family and friends

- possible risks and benefits the person associates with weight loss
- attitudes toward physical activity
- barriers, including time and financial limitations, that could frustrate weight loss efforts

Note that major depression is a poor prognostic indicator for weight loss (see page 111).

Encourage people who are not ready to lose weight and not at high risk to maintain their current weight by following as many of the components recommended for a healthy lifestyle as possible. Every attempt should be made to encourage the person to become physically active if they are currently sedentary. If they are already physically active, encourage them to increase their physical activity with a goal of 30 min of accumulated activity daily. Health care providers can help people at high risk identify the benefits and costs of losing weight. Factual information rather than pressure is more likely to increase readiness to change.

Weight loss is contraindicated for people

- with acute illness or in the terminal stages of an illness such as cancer
- with serious medical conditions that might be exacerbated by caloric restriction
- whose shortened life expectancy means that the benefits of weight loss and metabolic control will not be recognized (116,119)

Because of time limitations in my practice setting, I am unable to do a comprehensive nutrition assessment and provide guidance on meal planning in one visit— what should I do?

A comprehensive nutrition assessment is important to identify individual management goals and determine appropriate nutrition interventions. A nutrition assessment forms the basis for identifying practical lifestyle

changes to effectively improve health and diabetes outcomes. It is unrealistic to combine a nutrition assessment
and comprehensive education about individualized meal
planning in one visit. Here are several suggestions for what
you can do, especially if you are limited in time:

- Establish priorities—find out what the person wants to
  know, their interest level, and their willingness to make
  changes; keep in mind the nutrition education priorities
  such as awareness of carbohydrate and carbohydrate
  consistency, eating meals at regular times, and identifying a few eating behaviors to improve/change gradually
  over time
- Provide a diabetes self-care logbook and ask the patient
  to track food intake, physical activity, and blood glucose
  values for several days over the next week or two.
  Record keeping helps to increase awareness of current
  eating habits and physical activity levels and how they
  affect blood glucose levels. This information can also be
  used as a starting place for the follow-up visit.
- Combine an initial nutrition assessment with establishing personal goals and discussing some "beginning"
  changes in eating habits. Nutrition education resources
  available from the American Diabetes Association such
  as *The First Step in Diabetes Meal Planning* or *Healthy
  Food Choices* may help patients set goals and offer them
  ideas for healthier eating.
- Refer the patient to a dietitian with expertise in diabetes.
  They have more time allotted for appointments, a variety
  of visual aids and written educational materials, and experience assessing and integrating nutrition issues for people
  with other medical concerns in addition to diabetes.
- A nutrition assessment may be a reimbursable service.
  Federal and state laws have been passed over the past
  several years mandating reimbursement for diabetes self-
  management training and medical nutrition therapy.

Patient Education Goal Setting

How do I effectively set nutrition goals with a person who has diabetes?

Goal setting is a crucial part of diabetes self-management training. It is important to first differentiate between the different types of goals in diabetes. Diabetes management goals are clinical or metabolic outcomes of treatment intervention and may include clinical parameters such as glycated hemoglobin A1C, blood lipid levels, blood pressure, and body mass index (120). See pages 1–4 for the specific MNT goals that have been established (1). Standardized goals for education have also been established to help educators develop a successful education program. These goals acknowledge that diabetes self-management training occurs in different stages and is a continuous process. The American Diabetes Association has developed learning goals that correspond to the National Standards for Diabetes Self-Management Education (121,122).

Behavioral goals to assist in changing a person's lifestyle are also an important aspect of the management and education plan. They are less clinically focused but are individualized to patients' needs. The purpose of setting goals is to establish realistic target behaviors that can be used to evaluate patient success in making lifestyle changes. Goals are established by mutual agreement between the person with diabetes and the health care provider. This contributes to the likelihood that the patient will "own" the goals and become committed to the self-care behaviors that will enable him or her to reach and maintain them. To negotiate goals, providers need to be sensitive to the patient's need for flexibility and structure. It is important to respond to requests for guidance but also to encourage them to develop a realistic degree of independence in self-care. Below is a list of questions to elicit valuable information about where the patient is in their diabetes self-care and to help establish a lifestyle change plan (123).

- What behavior(s) would you like to change?
- What changes do you want to make to your current lifestyle?
- What are you willing to do right now?
- What obstacles do you see to making these changes?
- What benefits do you see as a result of making these changes?

The initial behavioral goals established with the patient should not be thought of as permanent. As time passes, their health, lifestyle, and attitudes will change. Goal set-

GOALS
Things I will do to improve my eating behavior

Check off each day you meet your goal.

Goal 1: Eat breakfast, lunch, and dinner every day.

M	T	W	T	F	S	S	M	T	W	T	F	S	S
M	T	W	T	F	S	S	M	T	W	T	F	S	S

Notes: _____

_____

_____

Goal 2: Eat five servings of fruits and vegetables every day.

M	T	W	T	F	S	S	M	T	W	T	F	S	S
M	T	W	T	F	S	S	M	T	W	T	F	S	S

Notes: _____

_____

_____

ting is a continuous process. A form or tool to assist the provider and the person with diabetes in goal setting is useful. The form should include a way to monitor or track daily progress. Each of the behavioral goals established should be specific and measurable. Starting with a small number of behavioral goals (perhaps one to three) that are achievable is also important in setting the patient up for success. The form on the previous page is an example of a tool to assist in setting goals for evaluating and improving lifestyle. Sample nutrition goals are also included in the form.

Educational Intervention

MEAL PLANNING APPROACHES

What is the latest thinking about nutrition plans in hospitals and long-term care facilities for patients with diabetes? Should we be using approaches such as no concentrated sweets, Exchange Lists, calorie levels, consistent carbohydrate, or carbohydrate counting?

Nutrition prescriptions that recommend meal plans such as no concentrated sweets, no sugar added, low sugar, or a "liberal diabetic diet" are not appropriate. These types of plans do not reflect the current diabetes nutrition recommendations and unnecessarily restrict sucrose. These approaches further perpetuate the myth that simply restricting sucrose-sweetened foods will improve blood glucose control (124).

The changes over the last decade in the American Diabetes Association (ADA) nutrition recommendations have forced dietitians and long-term care facilities to reconsider the way they are feeding people with diabetes. There is no such thing as an "ADA diet," but people use this term to refer to a predetermined calorie level with a specified percentage of carbohydrate, protein, and fat based on the Exchange Lists (124). Because the current nutrition recommendations of the ADA no longer endorse a specific type of meal plan or specified percentages of macronutrients, the "ADA diet" nutrition prescription is obsolete.

Standardized calorie-level meal plans have traditionally been used to plan meals for hospitalized patients. Just as there is no single nutrition prescription that meets the needs of every person with diabetes, there is no single meal planning system that is ideal for every hospital setting. There are a number of meal planning systems that can be used effectively in hospital settings. For example, patients with diabetes could be given a "regular" hospital menu based on the *Dietary Guidelines for Americans.* Another option is to use a "consistent carbohydrate meal plan." This system uses meal plans that incorporate a consistent carbohydrate content at each meal instead of setting a specific calorie level. A standard order could be developed for a "consistent carbohydrate meal plan" that represents ~1,800 calories with a distribution of 50% carbohydrate, 20% protein, and 30% fat. This would allow about 15 carbohydrate choices or servings/day, which could be distributed as four, five, and six servings of carbohydrate for breakfast, lunch, and dinner, respectively. After completing nutrition assessment to determine specific needs and preferences, a dietitian would then individualize the standard order. A task force of the ADA recommends that hospitals consider implementing the consistent carbohydrate meal plan approach (124).

What are the benefits of carbohydrate counting?

Carbohydrate counting is most often selected as a meal planning approach because it offers significant potential to improve blood glucose control. Both the Diabetes Control and Complications Trial (125) and the United Kingdom Prospective Study (126) have proven that good glycemic control prevents and delays diabetes complications. Carbohydrate counting was one of four meal-planning approaches used in the Diabetes Control and Complications Trial and was found to be effective in achieving glycemic control (127). The balance between carbohydrate and available insulin determines postprandial blood glucose response.

The American Diabetes Association nutrition recommendations encourage a focus on the total amount of carbohydrate rather than the type. Carbohydrate counting is the preferred meal planning approach used to implement intensive diabetes management, including continuous subcutaneous insulin infusion and multiple daily injections (1,15,128). In the Dose Adjustment for Normal Eating study, patients who learned from dietitians how to match insulin to carbohydrate experienced a greater decrease in glycated hemoglobin A1C and improved quality of life without a worsening of hypoglycemia (15). Focusing on carbohydrate is very useful to fine-tune diabetes control, reducing the incidence of hyperglycemia and hypoglycemia.

A second and very important benefit of carbohydrate counting is increased flexibility of food choices and timing of meals. By counting total carbohydrate, people with diabetes may choose the types of food they prefer at meals or snacks, often including highly varied combinations of foods, to reach the total carbohydrate goal for each meal or snack. This feature is highly attractive to people with diabetes, making carbohydrate counting a popular meal planning approach.

Third, carbohydrate counting is useful for all types of diabetes—type 1, type 2, or gestational diabetes. It can be individualized to fit any stage of life. Carbohydrate counting can be adjusted for individual needs and to meet the client's goals. For people familiar with the Exchange Lists, another widely used meal-planning approach, learning to make the change to counting carbohydrate is a very short step. Learning advanced carbohydrate counting takes practice and experience but offers great potential for more lifestyle flexibility.

When choosing a meal planning approach, what are some indicators that carbohydrate counting will be helpful?

Because the balance between carbohydrate and available insulin is the primary determinant of glucose concentrations, the more fully people understand carbohydrate counting, the better. People who use nutrition therapy only, or nutrition therapy and oral glucose–lowering agents, often improve their diabetes control using basic carbohydrate counting skills. Those who use intensive insulin regimens can benefit from applying advanced skills (129–131).

When helping people with diabetes choose a meal planning approach, carbohydrate counting becomes the obvious choice if the patient

- has heard or read about carbohydrate counting and asks to learn about it
- desires increased flexibility of food choices and timing of meals
- is frustrated with or confused by perceived dietary restrictions on sweets and desserts
- is excessively focused on avoiding sugar per se, without understanding that portions of all carbohydrate foods are equally important (e.g., "I only eat sugar-free pies")
- reads food labels for grams of sugar instead of total grams of carbohydrate
- has a nutrition history that shows frequent use of/preference for pasta, rice, potatoes, bread, ethnic foods (e.g., Italian, Mexican, oriental), sweets, and desserts
- avoids plant-based foods such as bread, potatoes, grains, fruits, and some vegetables because, "they will turn into sugar"

- reports unexplained problems with hypoglycemia, hyperglycemia, or both
- is unable to correctly identify single portion sizes of carbohydrate foods that they use regularly
- uses insulin, but makes no adjustments for hyperglycemia and/or hypoglycemia
- is looking for a fresh approach to diabetes meal planning
- has poor diabetes control (glycated hemoglobin A1C >8%)

What is basic carbohydrate counting vs. advanced carbohydrate counting?

Basic carbohydrate counting is the starting point of carbohydrate counting. Concepts include

- why count carbohydrate
- which foods contain carbohydrate
- what is a carbohydrate serving
- the need for portion control
- how to use food label information and other nutrition resources
- what is a free food
- the role of meat/meat substitutes and fat when counting carbohydrate

People learning basic carbohydrate counting can start by keeping records of food, physical activity, blood glucose monitoring, and medications, if used. Food records include the name of the food, portion sizes (household cups, ounces, teaspoons/tablespoons), and estimated carbohydrate content of each meal and/or snack.

Generally, several sets of at least 3 days of food records need to be collected over weeks or months. A dietitian knowledgeable about carbohydrate counting should evaluate each set of records for completeness and accuracy and to observe the patient's knowledge and skills for application. Food records provide a basis for establishing goals for carbohydrate intake at meals and, if desired, for snacks. Food records also provide a guide to additional teaching points to cover and possible problem-solving strategies. People implementing basic carbohydrate counting should be able to use a variety of educational resources to locate carbohydrate information, including the Nutrition Facts on a food label, food lists that identify carbohydrate counts, restaurant and fast food resources, and others, as needed. Teaching basic carbohydrate counting requires at least two 1-h visits over several weeks or months (131,132).

Advanced carbohydrate counting is appropriate primarily for people who use multiple daily injections or insulin pump therapy. Typically this includes people who have decided that they are willing to do what it takes to achieve a tighter level of blood glucose control—counting carbohydrates, checking blood glucose more often, being physically active, keeping food records, and making adjustments in their diabetes regimen based on their records. The purpose of advanced carbohydrate counting is to advance the patient's understanding of the relationships between food, medication, activity, and blood glucose (133).

Specifically, advanced carbohydrate counting is designed to teach pattern management and the use of insulin-to-carbohydrate ratios and correction factors. Pattern management refers to a three-step process (1):

1. identifying the patterns in blood glucose
2. identifying reasons for highs or lows
3. choosing an action plan to correct out-of-target blood glucose levels

Using insulin-to-carbohydrate ratios refers to the creation of a personal formula for figuring how much rapid-acting insulin to take to cover the carbohydrate in a meal or snack.

It is important to recognize and emphasize to people that advanced carbohydrate counting is not a do-it-yourself activity. People using advanced carbohydrate counting need to find and work closely with health care providers who are knowledgeable about this type of diabetes management.

What does it take for a person with diabetes to become skilled in carbohydrate counting?

Teaching checklists of the specific skills needed for both basic and advanced carbohydrate counting are as follows (131–134).

Basic carbohydrate counting skills

- understand that carbohydrate-containing foods are part of a healthy eating plan
- understand benefits of carbohydrate counting
- know what foods contain carbohydrate
- understand guidelines for incorporating sweets into food/meal plans
- measure (or estimate when in a situation where measuring is impossible) a serving of carbohydrate
- count servings, choices, or grams of carbohydrate
- know how many servings of carbohydrate to select for meals and snacks (if snacks are desired)
- understand portion control
- use portion control equipment: food labels, measuring equipment, and visual illustrations of portions
- have and use resources that list the carbohydrate content of foods and beverages
- know general guidelines for meat/meat substitutes and fat

Advanced carbohydrate counting skills

- master of all basic carbohydrate counting concepts
- explain basal (background) and bolus (mealtime) insulin
- understand insulin action

- understand insulin regulation for 24-h blood glucose control
- calculate insulin-to-carbohydrate ratio
- calculate insulin sensitivity factor and correction or supplemental doses
- determine mealtime insulin doses
- explain pattern management
- correct hypoglycemia
- correct hyperglycemia
- count carbohydrate and adjust insulin for special situations such as
  - meals with large servings of meat and/or fat
  - foods containing fiber
  - to minimize weight gain with improved glycemic control
  - restaurant foods
  - meals on vacations and holidays and in other people's homes
  - alcohol use
  - physical activity and exercise
  - sick days and stress

If there are no specific recommendations regarding the percentage or grams of carbohydrate, how should I start to determine the amount of carbohydrate a person should eat?

Ideally, a dietitian should be a member of the patient's diabetes management team. He or she would start with a comprehensive nutrition assessment to determine the amount of carbohydrate, types of carbohydrate, and consistency of carbohydrate from meal to meal/snack in the patient's current plan of eating. In addition, the dietitian should evaluate clinical parameters such as glycated hemoglobin A1C, body mass index and/or weight, and lipid levels to determine the recommended amount of carbohydrate in the meal plan (135).

However, in the real world, this is not always possible. If a dietitian is not available to individualize a meal plan, there is a simplified method that can be used as a starting place to determine carbohydrate, outlined in the table below (135).

Calculation of Carbohydrate (CHO) Servings (g CHO)	
To lose weight	
Women	2–3 servings CHO/meal (30–45 g)
Men	3–4 servings CHO/meal (45–60 g)
To control weight	
Women	3–4 servings CHO/meal (45–50 g)
Men	4–5 servings CHO/meal (60–75 g)
For active people	
Women	4–5 servings CHO/meal (60–75 g)
Men	4–6 servings CHO/meal (60–90 g)

What should my priorities be when I'm providing initial MNT to a newly diagnosed person with type 1 and type 2 diabetes?

A great place to start is to learn what the patient thinks or knows about food and diabetes, including their preconceptions or misconceptions. In addition, assess their interest and willingness to make changes in their current eating habits by asking what they would like to know about nutrition. To complement this, you should find out what the person typically eats and drinks for meals and snacks each day. Based on this information, you can determine whether the person with diabetes has a good understanding of healthy eating and the nutrition recommendations and priorities specific to the type of diabetes they have. To achieve the greatest success in promoting permanent changes in eating habits, start with what the patient is currently eating and set individualized goals for eating behavior change—as opposed to providing a calculated calorie prescription and giving a structured meal plan. To set them up for success, establish 1 or 2 relatively easy-to-achieve goals that will have an impact on blood glucose level (e.g., eat something in the first 2 h of the day, eat 25% less carbohydrate at dinner, walk for 10 min after eating a meal).

The nutrition education priority for people with type 1 diabetes is to adjust insulin based on carbohydrate intake at meals and mealtime blood glucose level. The nutrition education priorities for people with type 2 diabetes are to eat regular meals at regular times, spaced no more than 4 or 5 h apart and to establish a few, individualized eating behavior goals that make gradual changes in current lifestyle (see page 57).

TEACHING STRATEGIES

What can we do to maximize the effectiveness of MNT?

There is now evidence from several studies that nutrition therapy provided by dietitians can lower glycated hemoglobin A1C levels by ~2% and lower fasting plasma glucose by 50–100 mg/dl (13). Then why do we still hear comments that "diet fails"? Unfortunately, it is often the patient who is blamed for the failure—because they didn't lose weight or "follow the diet." Here are some common scenarios and reasons for why MNT may not be effective (136).

■ Providers tell the patient what to do by offering simplistic advice such as "lose a few pounds," "don't eat sugary foods," "don't drink soft drinks," "just eat less," and "stay away from fast food."
■ People with diabetes are given a preprinted diet sheet with a specified calorie level and a sample menu and told to follow it for an undetermined amount of time.

- The health care provider often does not aggressively promote MNT and physical activity as effective monotherapies.
- The pancreas is failing. Type 2 diabetes is a progressive disease (when diagnosed, the average person has already lost 50% of their beta cell function), and therapy needs to be intensified over time, specifically combining MNT and physical activity with medications such as oral glucose–lowering agents and/or insulin. MNT combined with physical activity is most effective with pre-diabetes (or metabolic syndrome) and during the initial phases of type 2 diabetes when insulin resistance is at its highest level. Dietitians and exercise therapists should have a key role when diabetes is first diagnosed and in the management of people at high risk for diabetes to prevent or delay the onset of the disease.

To maximize MNT effectiveness:

- Focus on lifestyle interventions that improve blood glucose control, lipids, and blood pressure instead of emphasizing weight loss.
- Focus on the specific nutrition interventions that will make the biggest difference—carbohydrate consistency, modification in the types and amount of fat, and portion control.
- Use food and blood glucose records to teach people with diabetes about food and glucose patterns and how they can be altered to improve their blood glucose control.
- Encourage physical activity—30 min of physical activity most days of the week. Suggest strategies such as using a pedometer to monitor activity (e.g., 10,000 steps equals 30 min of physical activity above and beyond normal activities of daily living).
- Make small, gradual changes in eating and physical activity behaviors; monitor progress at frequent follow-up visits (especially in the first 3 months—use phone or e-mail follow-up as needed), and revise as necessary to set patients up for success.

What advice can I offer to people with diabetes who struggle with overeating after their evening meal?

Recommending changes that people appear to ignore can be frustrating. Changes such as limiting evening snacks seems simple to understand and of obvious benefit. However, "simple to understand" is not the same as "simple to do." In the case of the after-dinner snacking habit, we see the following cycle in many individuals:

- in a hurry/not hungry so they skip breakfast
- too busy at work so lunch is skipped or they pick up a snack
- famished at the end of the day so they eat a huge dinner
- relax (and perhaps fall asleep) in front of the television with a large snack—often high in calories, sugar, and fat

For many people, eating is part of relaxing at the end of the day. By morning the cycle begins again. People tell us they are not hungry anyway. A common statement is, "I only eat when I am hungry, and I am not hungry until late afternoon. Besides, if I eat breakfast, I get even hungrier by lunch. Why waste calories by eating when you are not hungry? I will never lose weight that way."

Whether a person has type 1 or 2 diabetes and whatever his/her medication regimen, a large intake of calories before bed rarely contributes to optimal metabolic control. As a health care provider, this habit is hard to ignore, but so far your finest arguments have led to no positive results. What are some tactical options that might stimulate change and not ostracize the person?

Some possibilities to consider:

1. How often is it helpful to tell another adult what they have to do? What happens when you make a recommendation supported by rationale? Is the response any different?
2. Motivational interviewing describes a technique that avoids confrontation but asks questions about their personal goals and current behavior, working indirectly

to help the person see the discrepancy between what they say they want to accomplish and what they are doing. This may not create immediate change but perhaps stimulates interest in changing (137).

3. Would the individual be willing to try an experiment? What would happen if he or she ate a large snack for three nights in a row and then ate no snack for three nights in a row, recording food intake from dinner until morning and glucose levels at bedtime and in the morning? Discovering the problem rather than assuming it will result in a more acceptable solution (138).

4. Another experiment would be to check glucose levels after dinner. Sometimes people are hungry in the evening because their glucose is high after their largest meal of the day. One classic symptom of hyperglycemia is polyphagia. If there is inadequate insulin (injected or endogenous) available to cover the large meal, the glucose level may reach its highest level all day and the person could still actually be hungry. If someone overeats at dinner, why? Is it because they are overly hungry by the time they get home? Are they overmedicated? Do they eat too fast? Do they dine on carryout? Think of strategies to moderate the cause.

5. Can the person tell you whether or not they are really hungry after dinner? Or do they snack out of habit, boredom, or the need to do something with their hands? If together you can identify the impetus for eating, it opens the door for brainstorming alternatives. One person might like to do jigsaw puzzles, another might squeeze an exercise ball by the TV chair, and yet another might decide to schedule more evenings out. The possibilities are varied and limitless. Sometimes people think of solutions that the provider would never imagine, much less read in a book.

6. If for whatever reason the individual finds an evening snack essential, ask if there are snacks with more nutrients and fewer calories that would be satisfying. Some appreciate a list of snack options, including those avail-

able in single serving packaging. For others, agree on a calorie range and suggest that they find what is most satisfying within that range.

No single approach works or is appropriate for everyone. You and the person with diabetes can probably think of other strategies that better fit their individual situations.

Is it true that any food can be worked into a diabetes meal plan?

Many people request a list of foods they can and can't eat. At one time such lists constituted a meal plan, but research has expanded our understanding. The bad news is that meal planning for diabetes is not simple. The good news is that meal planning today is less restrictive and more effective than ever. People with diabetes can learn to include almost any food in their meal plan and still reach their treatment goals (2).

At the same time, overeating even the most nutritious of foods can interfere with treatment goals. The key is in the balance and variety, not the properties of individual foods. Ideally, meals include a measured amount of carbohydrate primarily from whole grains, fruits, and vegetables and with smaller amounts of protein and fat. Desserts, cheese, and pickles offer foods high in sugar, fat, and sodium, respectively, but all can enhance rather than hinder healthy eating if appropriately combined with other foods.

■ Frequency matters. It is what you do most of the time that counts. If occasional treats help one stay with the meal plan, in the long run, the treats may actually help improve outcomes.
■ Consider the volume and satisfaction level. Because the total amount of carbohydrate (and not the source) impacts glucose, chocolate cake can be substituted for a potato or candy for fruit. However, the volume of cake or candy will be much smaller. The patient must decide, "Is it worth it to me?"

- What goes with it? An ounce of cheese contains ~8 g fat and 100 calories. A slice of cheese that is added to a small hamburger creates a meal with 20–25 g fat. One slice of cheese in a plain bagel creates a meal with 8 g fat.
- Amount counts. A large dill pickle with 800 mg sodium would be hard to fit into a meal plan of <2,400 mg sodium/day. A couple slices of dill pickle on a hamburger with a piece of fruit provide a lunch well within the sodium restriction.
- The cut makes a difference. A 10-oz rib eye steak contains 1,000 calories. Ten oz of orange roughy is 250 calories. That is a calorie saving of 750 calories, equal to 2.5 h of walking for most people.
- Check out the preparation. A fish sandwich is breaded, fried, and typically served with tartar sauce. The fish sandwich usually contains more fat than a hamburger. Some salads offer more calories than a double cheeseburger.

One Hershey kiss after dinner is unlikely to elevate glucose levels, but a slice of sugar-free pie from the bakery will, due to its higher total carbohydrate content. The more people with diabetes learn about the effects of food on their blood glucose, the more they can incorporate a wide variety of favorite foods and still achieve their treatment goals.

Patient Follow-Up and Evaluation

To produce the best clinical and educational outcomes, how much and with what frequency do we need to provide MNT and/or diabetes self-management training (DSMT)?

It is impossible to give one absolute answer to this question. As all health care providers know, people with diabetes present with a wide array of skills, knowledge, motivation, needs, etc. The care and education of a person with diabetes must be individualized and provided consistently and continuously. However, the amount of care and frequency with which that care can be provided is currently constrained by private payors, Medicare, and Medicaid. Therefore, health care providers need to determine how they can maximize services for each person within the parameters of individual reimbursers.

Health care providers can find parameters to produce the best outcomes in the field-tested MNT nutrition practice guidelines (NPGs) for type 1, type 2, and gestational diabetes. These NPGs define the "best" nutrition care for people with diabetes. They are evidence based and describe diabetes nutrition care that results in positive health outcomes. They assist the health care provider in knowing what outcomes to evaluate to achieve positive results and at what intervals to schedule follow-up appointments. These NPGs are available for purchase as a CD-ROM online from the American Dietetic Association for a small fee at www.eatright.org.

It is well known that a single "diet instruction" or counseling session will not yield positive results for the vast majority of people with diabetes. In type 2 diabetes particularly, there is both a need for lifestyle changes and a natural disease progression. Helping people make lifestyle changes must be done over time with support and education. With the natural progression of type 2 diabetes comes the need to progress all aspects of management, from MNT and DSMT to medications to manage the metabolic parameters and possibly the chronic complications of diabetes.

The NPGs demonstrate that MNT for diabetes integrates nutrition with the medical and behavioral care of the individual. It is not just about tailoring a meal plan. MNT is also about reviewing blood glucose patterns and other metabolic parameters to provide feedback and recommendations to the patient and consulting with the health care provider if/when the diabetes management plan should be progressed. One study used in the development of the NPGs also showed that when the dietitian was actively involved in making decisions about interventions (e.g., nutrition prescriptions, the number of encounters needed, and medication changes) effectiveness of care was enhanced (4). It has been shown in two major diabetes prevention studies that consistent and continuous education and support is needed to help people make and maintain lifestyle changes (139,140).

In implementing MNT and/or DSMT for diabetes, it's important to use the four elements of care: assessment, goal setting, implementation, and evaluation. Consider these elements part of a continuous cycle to continually evaluate the patient's current status and assess what is and isn't working. Then set new goals and implement strategies that progress therapy to meet clinical targets and educational goals (141).

During the last several years, the American Association of Diabetes Educators has developed the National Diabetes Education Outcomes System (NDEOS). NDEOS is designed to support the educator's effort to track and report outcomes of DSMT. The goal of the project is to help educators develop a better understanding of what interventions work best in different populations and health care settings and to lead to an understanding of the best practices in DSMT (142). To learn more about NDEOS and its current status, see www.aadenet.org.

Physical Activity

Do people with diabetes need snacks for physical activity?

Most people with diabetes do not, but there are exceptions.

People with type 2 diabetes treated with MNT alone or in combination with an insulin sensitizer (e.g., metformin or glitazone) or α-glucosidase inhibitor do not risk hypoglycemia and rarely require snacks for increased activity. In fact, snacks add unnecessary calories, reducing the benefit of the activity.

For people with type 2 who take insulin or an insulin secretegogue, snacks are still rarely necessary if the physical activity is of mild-to-moderate intensity and is <30–45 min in duration. People who are physically active for more than an hour at high intensity levels are more likely to require glucose to prevent hypoglycemia during or after exercise. Each is an individual case, however, and the need for a snack is dependent on the duration and intensity of the activity and proximity of meals and medication peaks. Physical activity during a premeal blood glucose drop or during a peak in insulin action creates more risk for hypoglycemia and a potential need for additional glucose than does activity done 1–3 h after a meal (143).

For people with type 1 diabetes, if glucose levels are <100 mg/dl before the period of physical activity, additional glucose is recommended. If fasting glucose levels exceed 250 mg/dl with ketosis, troubleshoot the reason for hyperglycemia and delay the physical activity until ketones disappear. Without adequate insulin, hepatic glucose production can be stimulated and physical activity can further elevate rather than lower blood glucose (143).

People who have intensified their insulin therapy and calculate their insulin dose to match expected carbohydrate intake can add carbohydrate or reduce insulin to adjust for physical activity. If physical activity is unplanned or is moderate in intensity and short in duration, additional carbohydrate will reduce the risk for hypoglycemia. If physical activity is planned and longer than 2 h, reducing insulin is an alternative and recommended if weight reduction is a goal. Taking less rapid-acting insulin for the meal just prior to the activity or temporarily lowering the basal rate (for those on a pump) are other alternatives for reducing insulin for activity.

For people who have type 1 diabetes and are also serious athletes, adjustments to maintain glucose control during physical activity are more complex and require frequent monitoring to adjust extra carbohydrate (and/or reduce insulin) to maintain stable blood glucose during and after intense activity. An insulin pump works particularly well for these people because the basal rate can be lowered during and after the period of physical activity. The resources listed below provide more detailed recommendations for people with type 1 and type 2 diabetes involved in various activities. A summary of carbohydrate requirements for physical activity is provided in the table on pages 78–79.

Resources

Ruderman N, Devlin JT, Schneider SH, Kriska A (Eds.): *Handbook of Exercise in Diabetes.* Alexandria, VA, American Diabetes Association, 2002
Colberg S: *The Diabetic Athlete: Prescriptions for Exercise and Sports.* Champaign, IL, Human Kinetics, 2001
Diabetes Exercise and Sports Association at www.diabetes-exercise.org

How does physical activity decrease the risk of cardiovascular disease?

Physical activity decreases cardiovascular risk through a number of mechanisms (144):

- decreased blood pressure
- increased high-density lipoprotein cholesterol level
- decreased triglyceride level
- weight management
- increased fibrinolysis in response to thrombotic stimuli
- increased insulin sensitivity
- reduced susceptibility to serious ventricular arrythmias

Summary of Carbohydrate Requirements for Physical Activity

Treatment Mode/Preactivity Glucose	Preactivity Glucose Level	Physical Activity	Snack
Nutrition only or insulin sensitizer and/or α-glucosidase inhibitor		Any time or intensity	Rarely need extra carbohydrate
Type 2 Insulin or insulin secretegogue	Glucose <100 mg/dl	<30–40 min and mild-to-moderate activity or plan >60 min intense activity	Add 15 g carbohydrate/30–60 min activity; may need more if activity is before a meal or when insulin is peaking
	Glucose ≥100 but <250 mg/dl	Any time or intensity	Rarely need extra carbohydrate

			Add 15 g carbohydrate/ 30–60 min activity; may need more if activity is before a meal or when insulin is peaking
Intensive insulin regimen	Glucose <100 mg/dl	<30–40 min and mild-to-moderate activity or plan >60 min intense activity	
	Glucose ≥100 but <250 mg/dl		Need extra carbohydrate based on time and intensity of activity or reduce premeal or basal insulin rates
Type 1	Glucose ≥250 mg/dl with ketones	Physical activity is not recommended until ketones no longer detected	

- associated behavioral changes (e.g., smoking cessation, healthier eating, stress reduction)
- psychological benefits (e.g., decreased depression and anxiety)

Physical activity is also associated with changes in insulin sensitivity and lipid metabolism, events that are likely to have long-term effects on the development of cardiovascular complications. Aerobic activity benefits the cardiovascular system by decreasing heart rate at rest and during the activity, increasing stroke volume at rest and during the activity, and increasing cardiac output. Physical activity of moderate intensity is usually recommended for people with known coronary artery disease in the absence of ischemia or significant arrythmias.

Physical activity at regular intervals has been noted to decrease the risk of myocardial infarction. Sedentary individuals experience a higher relative risk of myocardial infarction after an episode of heavy exertion compared with individuals who engage in physical activity five or more times per week.

Sedentary lifestyles are closely associated with cardiovascular disease and obesity. Physical activity is a potent physiological stimulus of lipolysis, which results in the release of free fatty acids from triglycerides stored in fat for use as an energy source by muscle. Therefore, physical activity increases energy expenditure, which results in a negative calorie balance. Although physical activity alone may produce a 2–3% reduction in body mass index, it is most effective when used as an adjunct to medical nutrition therapy (119).

What types of physical activity improve cardiovascular risk factors?

Physical activity improves cardiovascular risk factors by increasing both heart rate and calorie expenditure (145). Walking is the most commonly prescribed activity and the most likely to be successful due to both safety and accessibility. A pedometer can be used to provide feedback concerning the number of steps or miles walked. Monitoring physical data is useful for shaping this behavior in small, simple steps. Individuals might begin by walking for 5–10 min 3 days per week and increasing the duration, frequency, and intensity of walking to the target level. The Diabetes Prevention Program intervention included 150 min of medium-intensity activity per week (139). Proponents of counting steps advocate 4,000 steps per day initially, increasing to 12,000 steps per day over 6 months to produce weight loss. The National Weight Control Registry, a longitudinal prospective study of individuals 18 years and older who have successfully maintained a 30-lb weight loss for a minimum of 1 year, reports participants engage in an average of 2,800 calories of physical activity weekly (146; see page 104).

All workouts should include 5- to 10-minute warm-up and cool-down periods. The warm-up increases core body temperature and prevents muscle injury; the cool-down prevents blood pooling in the extremities and facilitates removal of metabolic by-products. Physical activity should be performed on most days of the week or at least four times per week, with each session lasting between 30 and 60 min. This level of activity can be targeted to 60–80% of the maximum heart rate, which corresponds to 50–74% of the maximum oxygen consumption.

Physical activity of moderate intensity is generally recommended for the person with hypertension. Physical activity reduces blood pressure by 5–10 mmHg in some people, and its effects are usually noted within 10 weeks of training. Before starting a physical activity program, people with hypertension require adequate blood pressure control because some forms of physical activity cause acute increases in systolic pressure, an increase that may be exaggerated with diabetes. The blood pressure response to physical activity should be monitored initially, and adjustments in therapy should be made accordingly. High intensity exercises should be avoided because they can cause a significant pressor response.

The use of isometric (nonaerobic) activities for people with cardiovascular disease is prescribed less often than aerobic activity (144), but some studies suggest that properly designed resistance programs incorporating moderate levels of resistance and high repetitions may be safe for people with coronary artery disease, may favorably alter cardiovascular risk factors such as high-density lipoprotein cholesterol, and may improve insulin sensitivity.

Because both consistency and variety of physical activity are important for long-term success, people need to find activities they enjoy. Otherwise, new behaviors will likely be short lived. Thus, being physically active at a comfortable speed and intensity level are more important than pushing for high intensity. Prevention of injuries is critical also for the new behavior to persist.

Who needs a stress test before beginning a physical activity regimen?

People with both type 1 and type 2 diabetes have at least twice the morbidity and mortality related to myocardial infarction as the general population. In addition, many studies indicate that the incidence of asymptomatic coronary artery disease (CAD) or CAD associated with atypical symptoms is higher in the diabetes population. A 10% prevalence of occult, clinically-significant CAD in the typical clinic population with type 2 diabetes and without classic symptoms of ischemia is probably a conservative estimate (147). One of the most feared risks of initiating an exercise program is that of inducing sudden death secondary to an arrythmia or an ischemic event. This is most likely to occur when CAD is undiagnosed.

Therefore, before starting a physical activity program of moderate-to-high intensity (i.e., walking at rate of >3 miles/h), current American Diabetes Association recommendations for type 2 diabetes suggest that previously sedentary individuals >35 years of age or sedentary individuals of any age with duration of diabetes >10 years undergo stress testing (148). In addition, nephropathy, autonomic neuropathy, and peripheral vascular disease indicate the need for stress testing. Stress testing is most useful for people with a prior coronary event and people with nontraditional risk factors (e.g., autonomic neuropathy, peripheral vascular disease, proteinuria, and azotemia) (147).

Little is known about the risks of physical activity in people with type 1 diabetes, since most research is conducted in people with type 2 diabetes. Until additional information is available, anyone with the onset of type 1 diabetes in childhood or adolescence who is age ≥35 years or who has had diabetes for >15 years should be considered a high-risk patient.

Which is more effective for weight loss— physical activity or a calorie-restricted eating plan?

Physical activity is much more effective when used in combination with a calorie-restricted meal plan, rather than as a sole treatment modality. The combination of MNT and physical activity results in a greater degree of weight loss compared with MNT alone (149). This combination has also been shown to minimize the loss of lean body mass and the decrease in resting metabolic rate that accompanies weight loss (150); it produces a greater improvement in coronary heart disease risk factors than MNT alone—specifically, reductions in waist-to-hip ratio and triglycerides and increases in high-density lipoprotein cholesterol; and it can prevent diabetes (see page 139).

The benefits of an "MNT plus physical activity intervention," compared to an "MNT intervention," are more apparent in the maintenance of weight loss rather than initial weight loss. Physical activity is probably most effective for weight maintenance and improving glucose control.

The benefits of physical activity for people with diabetes can occur, however, without changes in body weight and body fat. Physical activity can improve glucose tolerance by reversing or decreasing insulin resistance and decreasing visceral abdominal fat. It also improves insulin sensitivity; however, that benefit is lost 48–72 h after physical activity ends, so maintaining insulin sensitivity requires regular activity. Both aerobic and muscle-strengthening physical activity can contribute to improved glucose control.

Are intermittent or short bouts of physical activity really effective for people with diabetes?

Accumulating physical activity over the course of the day in several short sessions, such as a 10-minute walk three times/day, has been included in recent recommendations from the Centers for Disease Control and the American College of Sports Medicine, as well as the National Institutes of Health Consensus Development Conference on Physical Activity and Health (151).

Intermittent physical activity can be especially effective in people with type 2 diabetes who have higher levels of insulin resistance, especially when diagnosed. Because of the delay in the first phase of insulin release, people with type 2 diabetes often have higher postprandial glucose levels and a slower return to target glucose levels. Doing some type of physical activity for 10–15 min after meals can significantly reduce the postprandial glucose level.

Unfit people with diabetes may have difficulty sustaining activity for longer durations or may feel that long bouts of physical activity are boring. The energy expenditure of multiple short bouts of physical activity throughout the day is similar to that of a traditional longer bout of activity. It provides the same health-related benefits and can also assist with long-term weight loss (152). Developing a pattern of short bouts of physical activity may also empower the person with diabetes to identify barriers, such as time, that might otherwise inhibit the activity. It also has the advantage of letting the person choose convenient times throughout the day to perform mini-bouts of vigorous physical activity—although, for the person with type 2 diabetes, the best time to complete the short bout of physical activity is after a meal.

Why is physical activity so important?

Cardiorespiratory fitness is shown to reduce all-cause mortality across all categories of body composition. One large cohort prospective study (25,925 men, age 30–83 years) observed no elevated mortality risk in obese men if they were fit, regardless of their percentage of body fat, and lean men had increased longevity only if they were physically fit, regardless of their body composition or risk factor status (153). Unfit lean men had double the risk of all-cause mortality compared to fit lean men and had a higher risk of all-cause and cardiovascular mortality than did men who were fit and obese. Similar results have recently been reported in a cohort of women; low cardiorespiratory fitness was a stronger predictor than body mass index of all-cause mortality in women (154).

In the Lee et al. study, a cohort included 1,263 men with type 2 diabetes at baseline; 534 (42%) were in the low-fit category and 729 (58%) in the fit category (155). Men who were physically inactive had an adjusted risk for mortality that was 1.7-fold higher than those who were physically fit. Furthermore, a cohort subgroup of 593 men developed impaired fasting glucose and 149 developed type 2 diabetes (156). The risk for diabetes was 3.7-fold higher in the low-fitness group than for the men in the high-fitness group.

There is also a growing body of evidence indicating that exercise without weight loss improves insulin sensitivity (157). Encourage people at risk for diabetes in addition to those with diabetes to perform regular physical activity, such as brisk walking, for 30–60 min on most days of the week. Not only does physical activity decrease risk for all-cause mortality and diabetes and improve insulin sensitivity, it also improves overall health and well-being. If the person with diabetes has not been successful with weight loss through eating fewer calories and/or fat, perhaps they can be successful in improving other risks for coronary heart disease through increased physical activity.

When discussing the benefits of being physically active, people commonly tell me, "I don't have time!" or "I don't like to exercise!" How can I get people interested in being physically active and help them to stick with it?

- Ask them to purchase and wear a pedometer to increase their awareness of how much physical activity they accumulate throughout the day and to provide an incentive to increase physical activity. They can compare their actual number of steps/day with a goal of 10,000 steps/day, which is equivalent to 30 min of physical activity above and beyond normal activities of daily living (158).
- Suggest that they keep a food/exercise logbook. A logbook can help them identify patterns and provide feedback on progress.
- Start with individualized goals regarding the type of activity, frequency, and duration and then progress to recommended levels (e.g., a 10-minute walk to the mailbox 5 times/week).
- Think of ways to increase physical activity through activities of daily living (e.g., take the stairs instead of the elevator, walk the dog, vacuum the floor, park your car at the far end of the parking lot, mow the lawn).

- Suggest creative options such as intermittent exercise (e.g., 10-minute walk after meals).
- Assist in finding a physical activity that they would enjoy (e.g., walking is most popular for people with diabetes who are not regular exercisers).
- Have patients think about physical activities that would
  - be fun: any kind of dancing; water aerobics; team sports such as volleyball, basketball, and tennis
  - be doable: move around during TV commercials; perform chair aerobics; work with a physical therapist on an individualized exercise evaluation
  - allow them to accomplish more than one activity at once: read, watch TV, or listen to a music or book tape while using an exercise bike or treadmill; biking with family members

Medication

What are the nutrition implications of the different oral agents?

There are five categories of oral agents listed in the table on pages 88–89. Glucophage and the thiazolidinediones (TZDs) are identified as insulin sensitizers. Sulfonylureas and meglitinides stimulate increased insulin production. Different diabetes medications taken alone have implications for meal planning (1; see table on pages 88–89).

How important is it to match the eating plan with the insulin regimen?

Insulin therapy is most effective when glucose from digested food and insulin reach the bloodstream at the same time. The insulin action curves of rapid-acting, short-acting, intermediate-acting, and long-acting or basal insulins are all different, as their names suggest (159).

Oral Agent	Side Effects	Nutrition Implication
Metformin	Gas, bloating, diarrhea Tends to blunt appetite May see 2- to 5-kg weight loss Improves lipid profile Risk for lactic acidosis increases with heavy alcohol intake Associated with reduced B_{12} levels	Minimized if eaten with or after food or if started on low dose. Optimal absorption on empty stomach Supports weight loss efforts Assess alcohol consumption Assess B_{12} status in elderly and others at risk for inadequate absorption
TZDs	Associated with mild-to-moderate edema and weight gain May promote return of ovulation and/or reduce effectiveness of oral contraceptives Well absorbed without regard to meals	May require diuretics to reduce fluid retention which could nudge glucose levels upward May benefit from sodium restriction Risk of pregnancy

α-Glucosidase inhibitors	Delays carbohydrate absorption from the gut by interfering with digestion of starch and sucrose.	Take with first bite of food. If combined with oral glucose–lowering agent that can cause hypoglycemia, use glucose or milk (not sucrose or fructose) to treat hypoglycemia
	Gas, bloating, diarrhea	Avoid taking with other drugs or conditions with similar side effects
		Minimize by starting on low dose
Sulfonylureas	May cause hypoglycemia	Avoid delaying or skipping meals; may need to lower dose or change type of medication
	Weight gain	Consider alternate agent as initial therapy if overweight
	Takes longer to be absorbed	Take 30 min before meal
Meglitinides	Slight risk for hypoglycemia	Take within 30 min of each meal
		Allows flexibility in timing of meals and exercise
	Short acting (half-life 1–1.5 h) to target postprandial glucose	May need to limit or avoid snacks to prevent rise in glucose between meals

Adapted from White JR, Campbell RK: Pharmacologic therapies for glucose management. In *Diabetes Management Therapies. A CORE Curriculum for Diabetes Education.* 5th ed. Franz MJ, Ed. Chicago, American Association of Diabetes Educators, 2003, p. 136

Relative Insulin Action by Insulin Type

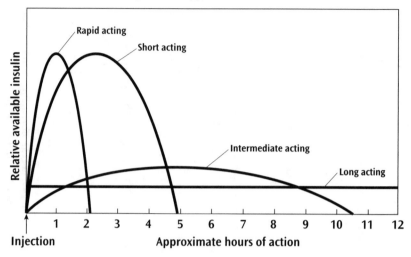

Rapid-acting insulin begins to work in 5 min; it should be taken within 15 min before eating, or during or after food intake. Rapid-acting insulin provides coverage for the food that immediately follows but peaks in 1 h and fades within 3–5 h so that little is available to cover between-meal snacks. People taking rapid-acting insulin are likely to have elevated glucose levels at the next meal if they snack between meals. However, because mealtime insulin is relatively short acting, the person with diabetes is at less risk for hypoglycemia between meals and can choose to eat at a time most convenient for his or her schedule.

A common insulin regimen is a rapid- or short-acting insulin taken in combination with an intermediate-acting insulin. Combined, the intermediate-acting insulin influences the action of the rapid- or short-acting insulin, resulting in a bimodal curve with the first peak intended to cover breakfast and the second to cover the midday meal. If regular (short-acting) insulin is used, the best match between food and insulin occurs if the insulin is injected

30 min before the meal begins. The effective duration of this combination injection is 10–16 h.

Premixed combination insulins, such as 70/30 insulin, a combination of 70% NPH (intermediate acting) and 30% rapid- or short–acting insulin, are convenient and require fewer injections per day and use of snacks. However, they offer less flexibility and cannot accommodate day-to-day variability in food intake or timing of meals. For many, the 70/30 insulins provide more insulin than needed in the late morning and require a snack to avoid hypoglycemia before lunch, especially when physical activity is added. If the insulin dose before the evening meal is high enough to cover the meal, some people require an evening snack to avoid hypoglycemia during the night. Snacks can undermine weight-loss efforts.

A switch to a long-acting basal insulin, such as glargine, with rapid-acting insulin at meals changes insulin action time and the timing of food to match it. Basal insulin is peakless and intended to cover only glucose produced by the liver and other background insulin needs. People who switch from a two-injection 70/30 regimen to one that uses basal insulin plus rapid-acting insulin before meals find they can be more flexible about when they eat and can match carbohydrate intake with an appropriate dose of rapid-acting insulin for greater flexibility with food content, with the bonus of improved glucose levels. This regimen requires injections 4 times/day (one injection of rapid-acting insulin at each meal and usually glargine once a day at bedtime).

Reevaluate each patient's individualized meal plan anytime there is a change in the medication regimen (2). You can maximize the benefits of the newer treatment options when you know how different medications, food, and the physiology of diabetes interact.

I frequently receive referrals to teach carbohydrate counting to an individual planning to use an insulin pump. What is different about working with a person using an insulin pump versus someone using multiple daily injection (MDI) therapy?

Very little. Advanced carbohydrate counting is appropriate for both MDI and pump therapy (131, 160). Both regimens make provisions for basal insulin coverage and boluses to cover meal carbohydrate, usually with rapid-action insulin. To take advantage of the benefits of these regimens, a person should learn all the skills of basic and advanced carbohydrate counting (see pages 62–65).

In advanced carbohydrate counting, the mealtime insulin dose is determined based on the amount of carbohydrate the person plans to (or has) eaten and any correction dose to adjust for premeal hyper- or hypoglycemia. Therefore, it is necessary to count carbohydrate accurately.

Carbohydrate may be counted in grams (total carbohydrate as read from the nutrition facts label) or in servings (choices) each equal to about 15 g carbohydrate. However, counting grams is more accurate because one carbohydrate serving, according to the Exchange Lists, may vary from 11 to 20 g. A typical 4–carbohydrate serving meal would then contain about 60 g carbohydrate. Therefore, someone counting servings, even if carefully measured, could actually be consuming from 44 to 80 g carbohydrate. Such a difference would influence mealtime insulin dosing. Patients counting carbohydrates need to

■ know the carbohydrate content of the foods they eat. Foods with nutrition fact labels are relatively easy. It may take some time to locate food composition data for produce and restaurant foods.
■ accurately estimate portions of various foods. It takes time to measure portions of foods eaten at home with labels. More difficult is training the eye to see the difference between a 15-, 25-, and 30-g apple or the portion

of mashed potatoes versus baked potato or corn on the cob at a restaurant.

■ learn how to calculate and use an insulin-to-carbohydrate ratio and a correction factor to adjust for high or low glucose.

■ monitor glucose frequently enough to evaluate the effectiveness of insulin-to-carbohydrate ratios and correction or sensitivity factor.

■ keep records to identify patterns in food, insulin, and blood glucose. Circling highs in blue and lows in red is one way of spotting patterns for management purposes.

People proficient with advanced carbohydrate counting may enjoy increased flexibility and still maintain good control, whether with MDI or a pump.

Features of an insulin pump that may affect food intake include the following.

■ Having the ability to adjust basal rates on the pump may change the insulin-to-carbohydrate ratios.

■ An injection is not required for snacks—a convenience as well as an opportunity to add extra calories and gain weight.

■ There is an option to adjust for high-fat meals or a social evening of appetizer grazing using the bolus options. These features program the pump to deliver bolus insulin over time.

■ There is the option to lower basal insulin rather than add a snack for exercise.

Pattern Management

Why might someone have an insulin reaction less than an hour after a large meal?

Anyone who takes a set amount of insulin and varies the composition of his or her meals is likely to experience swings in glucose levels. If he or she takes the usual insulin dose and eats a very low–carbohydrate meal, like a steak and tossed salad, it is possible to consume 1,000–1,500 calories or more and still experience hypoglycemia when the insulin peaks in 1–2 h because of the inadequate carbohydrate intake (161).

People with diabetes may also experience hypoglycemia if regular or rapid-acting insulin is taken so soon that the insulin is peaking before the food is digested. This happens when eating is interrupted by a phone call or delayed at a busy restaurant. An example is a person who takes his insulin in the car just before entering a fast food restaurant and then discovers that he has no money and is not able to eat. Much too frequently, people with diabetes take their insulin at home before going (and driving) to a restaurant (159).

Planning for such times requires more common sense than medical science but does highlight the benefit of having patients understand the rationale for recommendations (e.g., how their medications interact with food) and the need to consider nonroutine circumstances.

How important is it to space meals and eat them on time?

It is helpful to space meals and eat them on time. How close to eating at the exact same time each day depends on a number of factors, including personal preference, scheduled activity, medications, and type of diabetes.

With or without diabetes, most people benefit from distributing food and carbohydrate intake throughout the day. Breakfast is the first step, one that is difficult for many. The benefits of breakfast for schoolchildren has led to programs to provide breakfast at school (162). More recently, researchers announced that eating breakfast may help lower the risks of obesity, insulin resistance, and diabetes. In a group of 2,681 young adults, those who ate breakfast daily developed obesity and insulin resistance at a rate 35–50% lower than those who did not eat breakfast during the 8 years of the study (163). Eating breakfast is associated with successfully maintaining weight loss (see pages 104–106).

Another study found that given equal calorie intake, eating three or nine times a day made no difference in glucose control (164). However, in a study of adolescents, the more frequently the subjects ate, the more calories, carbohydrate, and sugar they consumed (165). People trying to lose weight may have more difficulty limiting calories with multiple snacks. However, if the time between meals is too long, the temptation may be to consume more food faster with less discretion than if they ate regularly and came to the table less famished. Optimal timing still depends on individual preferences and experience of hunger, fatigue, and glucose levels. Blood glucose monitoring results provide useful information to guide decisions.

The number of meals and snacks and mealtime flexibility depend on the medication regimen. Longer-acting insulin or insulin secretegogues mandate a more regular eating schedule than shorter-acting ones. For example, NPH insulin peaks in 4–12 h and lasts up to 24 h. If taken at breakfast, eating lunch on time or adding a morning snack is required to avoid hypoglycemia. Rapid-acting insulin or meglitinide work quickly and the risk of decreased blood glucose with exercise or a delayed meal is much lower, so mealtime is quite flexible as long as the medication is taken close to the meal. In many cases, such as with kids or when eating out, it's probably better to recommend that people take their rapid-acting insulin after they have determined approximately how much carbohydrate is in their meal and when the food is actually in front of them. Similarly, with α-glucosidase inhibitors, timing is flexible, but the medication is only effective if taken within a few minutes of the start of the meal. There is no special reason beyond those for the general diabetes population to eat regular meals if using metformin or thiazolidinediones, alone or in combination, because they cannot cause low blood glucose.

Why should we teach people with type 2 diabetes who take insulin how to adjust insulin using correction bolus doses of rapid-acting insulin based on mealtime glucose level and estimated carbohydrate intake (pattern management)?

People with type 2 diabetes who require insulin, alone or in combination with oral glucose–lowering medication, to reach their target blood glucose level have usually progressed in the disease process from the initial stage of insulin resistance and relative insulin deficiency to becoming insulin deficient. Using a more intensive insulin regimen and teaching blood glucose pattern management to make self-adjustments in insulin, eating, and/or physical activity can assist in fine-tuning blood glucose levels and reaching target blood glucose goals (166,167).

The decision to use this approach should not be based on the person's type of diabetes but, rather, on their desire for improved blood glucose levels, their need for flexibility, and their willingness to do the "extra work"—that is, regular, frequent blood glucose monitoring, 3–4 insulin injections/day, and making careful, individualized decisions about the doses of mealtime rapid-acting insulin based on glucose levels and carbohydrate intake. If the person with diabetes is not reaching glucose goals with their current diabetes regimen and expresses interest, certainly this more intensive type of regimen should be considered (168).

Why is the combination of an insulin-to-carbohydrate ratio/correction factor approach better for calculating mealtime insulin doses than a sliding scale approach?

A sliding scale approach to adjustment of insulin is retrospective or reactive, in that it provides insulin, which should be working prospectively over the next few hours, to treat an elevated blood glucose level that has already occurred. In addition, using a sliding scale approach does not factor in the amount of carbohydrate that is consumed at the meal when the insulin bolus is taken. For these two reasons, the sliding scale approach should no longer be used. It results in "chasing" blood glucose levels and often, a roller coaster ride of high and low blood glucose levels throughout the day. A sliding scale adjustment is often used to correct a single blood glucose value at a particular moment in time. For example, if a patient's blood glucose level is 180 mg/dl (50 mg over their target), they may be instructed to take 1 extra unit of insulin. If the glucose level is 100 mg/dl over their target, they would take 2 extra units of insulin, and so on. This is a quick-fix remedy and not a problem-solving approach (166,167).

A combination insulin-to-carbohydrate ratio/correction factor approach to insulin dosing is prospective or proactive in that it involves individualizing the insulin dose based on the mealtime blood glucose level and estimating the amount of carbohydrate to be eaten at the meal. This approach allows the person to treat high blood glucose levels several times a day and to calculate an insulin dose that also covers the carbohydrate they eat. For example, if a patient estimated their usual carbohydrate intake at lunch to be 75 g, they would divide this by the number of units of premeal insulin they usually take. That is, if they would usually take 5 units of premeal insulin, they would divide 5 into 75 and figure an insulin-to-carbohydrate ratio of 1:15. For every 15 g carbohydrate, they would take 1 unit insulin; for a 75-g carbohydrate meal, they would take 5 units insulin before the meal. The next step would be to combine the insulin-to-carbohydrate ratio with a correction factor. The correction factor involves individualizing the insulin dose based on the patient's premeal blood glucose level. The formula for this correction factor is 1,500 (short-acting insulin) or 1,800 (rapid-acting insulin) divided by the patient's total daily insulin dose. If a patient took 30 total units of insulin per day, their correction factor would be 60 (1,800/30 = 60). This is the mg/dl the blood glucose level will decrease with 1 unit of insulin. If a patient had a prelunch meal blood glucose of 190, they would take 1 extra unit of insulin to bring their blood glucose down to target range (<130 mg/dl). So, they would take the 5 units of insulin to cover the 75 g carbohydrate and 1 unit insulin to correct the high premeal blood glucose or a total of 6 units of insulin.

What strategies can be used to determine an optimal medication plan that considers patients' food habits, preferences, and lifestyle?

The availability of various oral glucose–lowering medications and numerous insulins allows people with diabetes and their health care providers to chose a medication regimen that matches the physiological disturbances of diabetes, the stage of diabetes, and the person's food habits and lifestyle. Choosing a medication plan without the input from the person about their food habits and lifestyle can make adherence more difficult for them and lead to frustration on the part of the health care provider. Gathering this information also gives the health care provider insights into the quality and quantity of the person's food intake, cultural preferences, and the elements of their lifestyle they need to—and are willing to—change.

The following questions can help health care providers obtain information about a person's food habits and lifestyle. They also provide an opportunity to assess and elicit a person's interest in making lifestyle changes and to set an honest and positive tone for working together in a partnership.

1. Can you describe the average weekday and weekend day in your life? Include what you do, the times you eat, what you eat, and where you eat. Include if/when

you exercise, what type of physical activity you do, and how much time you spend doing it.

2. How does your schedule vary from day to day, weekday to weekend? Describe your hours of work, activity level, and times of your meals and snacks.

3. Do you eat snacks between meals? If so, why? What foods do you eat and when?

4. What is your assessment of your eating habits? Are there behaviors you would like to change?

5. What aspects of a healthy eating plan are most difficult for you to follow?

6. What are you willing/able and unwilling/unable to change about your eating habits and meal schedule?

7. Do you currently have problems with hunger, low blood glucose reactions (what time of day, what blood glucose levels), high blood glucose levels (what time of day, what blood glucose levels), and/or weight gain?

8. What are you interested in learning that will help you better manage your diabetes?

For instance, a woman with newly diagnosed type 2 diabetes who is overweight is put on a sulfonylurea. In addition, she is encouraged to lose weight by decreasing food intake and starting a walking program. She begins making these lifestyle changes and her blood glucose levels are lower. In fact, two to three weeks later, she gets lightheaded and hungry on several afternoons. She feels better after eating a few crackers with juice. But having to eat this snack frustrates her because it forces a higher intake of calories and interferes with weight loss.

It is difficult enough for people with type 2 diabetes to lose weight and control their hunger without having the medication work against their efforts. Choosing an insulin sensitizer (e.g., metformin or a glitazone), rather than a sulfonylurea, may more effectively treat the major physiologic problems of early type 2 diabetes—insulin resistance and hepatic gluconeogenesis—without the risk of and need to treat hypoglycemia.

Here's another example. A woman with type 1 diabetes typically eats three meals a day—a small breakfast, medium lunch, and large dinner. The timing of these meals varies due to work and family obligations. She has been encouraged to eat an afternoon and evening snack to prevent hypoglycemia but finds snacks a bother. Her insulin regimen is the same each day: NPH and aspart before breakfast, aspart at dinner, and NPH before bed. She has at least three or four episodes per week of hypoglycemia, in afternoons and/or during the night. She is tired of having to eat when she doesn't want to eat to prevent or treat hypoglycemia.

A regimen of long-acting insulin (glargine) with doses of rapid-acting insulin at each meal based on the current blood glucose level and the amount of carbohydrate in the meal would fit her lifestyle and needs more adequately. This approach can help avoid some hypoglycemia, decrease undesired food intake, and increase flexibility with her meal times and amount of carbohydrate.

Obesity/Weight Maintenance

What is the current thinking on the use of high-protein, low-carbohydrate diets for people with diabetes?

Controversies about popular fad diets abound. During the last half of 2002, the media promoted an ongoing dialogue about fad diets that began with a July 7 article in *The New York Times* (169). This article suggested that the recommendation to eat foods low in fat—long lauded by government and many health organizations, including the American Diabetes Association—has triggered the US obesity epidemic. The article led to spin-off articles in many nutrition and health newsletters that portrayed an image of nutrition experts being in a tug-of-war over the best advice (170,171). Additional fuel was added to the fire after a Duke University study was presented at the annual American Heart Association meeting in November 2002 suggesting that the low-carbohydrate, high-fat Atkins diet could improve blood lipids. Consumers and health care professionals have been left confused trying to sort fact from fiction.

The truth is that the jury is still out on the Atkins diet and high-protein, low-carbohydrate meal plans, particularly for people with diabetes. A recent one-year, randomized trial compared high-protein, low-carbohydrate diets to a conventional low-calorie, high-carbohydrate, low-fat diet (172). Researchers reported 4% greater weight loss at 6 months in the study group compared to the conventional diet, but differences were not significant at one year. Adherence was poor and attrition was high in both study groups. Authors concluded that longer and larger studies are required to determine long-term safety and efficacy of such diets. Another recent systematic review of the efficacy and safety of low-carbohydrate eating plans concluded there is insufficient evidence to make recommendations for or against the use of low-carbohydrate foods, particularly among participants age >50 years, for use longer than 90 days, or for eating plans of ≤20 g carbohydrate/day (173). Also, authors concluded that more careful studies of people with and without diabetes and with and without lipid abnormalities are needed to more fully describe the effects of lower-carbohydrate eating plans on lipid and glycemia indices and ketogenesis.

Research supported by the National Institutes of Health is underway that should provide more objective data on the long-term effects of such eating plans. Experts agree that there are no simple answers or quick fixes to the difficult issue of weight management in the US. It is true that high-protein, low-carbohydrate eating plans produce substantial initial weight loss—partly due to fluid loss and partly because people end up eating fewer calories due to limited choices and the effect of ketones to decrease appetite. However, these eating plans do not appear effective for long-term weight maintenance (174). Major concerns about the safety of using them in people with diabetes exist, including potential progression of cardiovascular disease (175), cancer (176), osteoporosis (177), gout, and renal disease (175,177). Nutrition concerns include loss of water-soluble vitamins with diuresis; inadequate fiber, calcium, and B vitamins; and depletion of glycogen stores.

The Albert Einstein College of Medicine in New York City has initiated the first national Controlled Carbohydrate Assessment Registry Bank Study (CCARBS), which tracks the food intake and weight patterns of individuals following a controlled-carbohydrate lifestyle over a period of several years. CCARBS data will also be used to study the lipid patterns of registry participants. For more information, see the CCARBS Study web site: http://ccarbs.aecom.yu.edu.

Experts agree that people with diabetes should

- cut back on saturated (and *trans*) fat. This includes hamburgers, French fries, pizza, ice cream, and sweets, and snack foods made with butter, shortening, stick margarine, or hydrogenated oil.
- monitor total carbohydrate intake and avoid excesses. Consistent amounts of carbohydrate at meals and snacks and/or adjustment of medications to cover planned carbohydrate intake promotes improved blood glucose.
- individualize weight loss strategies to problem solve particular food behaviors. Some may find it easier to reduce calories by cutting back on bread, pasta, rice, potatoes, and sweets, whereas others choose to cut back on fried foods, fast foods, snack foods, salad dressing, and mayonnaise. Including at least five servings of vegetables and fruits plus two to three low-fat dairy products is recommended for good nutrition. Attention to portions consumed is needed by all.

Until more evidence becomes available about the safety and effectiveness of high-protein, low-carbohydrate eating plans, they should not be recommended to people with diabetes.

What are the best indicators for assessing health risk from obesity?

Obesity researchers have published and promoted the use of evidence-based, practical guidelines to educate health care providers in treating obesity as a medical disorder (119). The guidelines support classification and assessment of obesity as an important component of the person's medical care. The clinical guidelines recommend measuring body mass index (BMI) and waist circumference as "vital signs" for evaluation of the person who is obese.

BMI has replaced ideal body weight as a criterion for assessing obesity because it correlates with body fat, morbidity, and mortality. BMI can be calculated quickly or extracted from a BMI chart in a busy clinical setting. Furthermore, recommendations for the treatment of obesity are based on BMI. Additionally, the World Health Organization Obesity Task Force developed a classification system for obesity according to BMI that has been adopted by the Expert Panel on the Identification, Evaluation and Treatment of Overweight and Obesity in Adults, a group assembled by National Heart, Lung, and Blood Institute of the National Institutes of Health (119,178).

Waist circumference is another important measure of obesity risk, as it indicates visceral abdominal fat. Evidence suggests that abdominal fat carries a higher health risk than peripheral fat, and that the visceral fat component correlates most strongly with increased risk (179). A high-risk waist circumference is accepted to be >35 inches for women and >40 inches for men. Waist circumference may have additional value in the elderly, in whom decreased muscle mass contributes to underestimation of obesity-related risk by BMI alone.

			Classification of Overweight and Obesity by BMI, Waist Circumference, and Associated Disease Risks	
	BMI	**Obesity Class**	**Disease Risk* Relative to Normal Weight Waist Circumference**	
			Men <40 in	>40 in
			Women <35 in	>35 in
Underweight	<18.5		—	—
Normal	18.5–24.9		—	—
Overweight	25.0–29.9		Increased	High
Obesity	30.0–34.9	I	High	Very high
	35.0–39.9	II	Very high	Very high
Extreme	>40	III	Extremely high	Extremely high

*Disease risk for type 2 diabetes, hypertension, and cardiovascular disease.

What is the National Weight Control Registry (NWCR), and what have we learned from it?

The NWCR, initiated in 1993 by obesity experts at the University of Pittsburgh and the University of Colorado, is the largest set of data ever collected about successful weight maintainers (180). The purpose of the registry was to use quantitative measures to describe weight loss and weight maintenance strategies and to categorize groups within the larger sample. The intent of developing the registry also was to collect data that could be used to respond to the general skepticism and pessimism among health care providers about the efficacy and safety of medical treatment of obesity. Developers of the registry wished to refute the all-too-often quoted statistic from 1959 that 95% of those who initially lose weight will regain their weight.

Entry criteria for the NWCR requires participants to be >8 years old, to have lost at least 30 lb, and to have kept the weight off for at least 1 year. Participants have been, in large part, recruited through newspaper, magazine, and television releases. Currently, nearly 3,000 participants are included in the registry. Participants significantly exceed minimum criteria for entry into the registry, having lost an average total of 71 lb and kept their weight off for an average of 6 years.

A variety of methods to lose weight were used by registry participants. Thirty-six percent report having lost weight on their own; 64% lost weight with assistance (181). Weight loss methods included commercial programs, self-help groups, dietitians, psychologists, liquid diets, and combinations of the above.

Eating behaviors reported by the successful weight maintainers include:

- 93.6% restrict certain foods (e.g., high-sugar and high-fat foods)
- 78% eat breakfast daily
- 50% rely heavily on portion control
- 39% limit their dietary fat intake
- 36% count calories
- 30% count fat grams
- 16% use the Exchange Lists system (182)

Registry participants report an average intake of 1,400 calories per day and an average of 2,800 calories of physical activity expenditure per week (albeit research has shown people typically underestimate food intake and overestimate physical activity). Participants also weigh themselves regularly and limit eating out in restaurants to less than three times per week.

Data show that, regardless of the methods used for weight loss, with one exception, strategies for weight maintenance are similar (183). People who have undergone surgical treatment of obesity report higher intake of dietary fat, lower intake of carbohydrate and protein, and lower physical activity (184).

Nearly 77% of registry participants reported that there was a triggering event or incident that preceded their successful weight loss. Three types of triggers were identified: 1) medical (e.g., heart attack), 2) emotional (e.g., "my husband left me, and his lawyer told me it was because I was fat"), and 3) lifestyle (e.g., a child's wedding, 25th anniversary, etc).

The NWCR provides evidence that weight loss achieved by limiting dietary fat and calories and increasing physical activity can be maintained for long periods. Although the actual prevalence rate of successful weight loss and maintenance remains unclear, the NWCR data show clearly that some individuals are highly successful at losing weight and keeping it off. For more information about the NWCR and recruiting participants for this registry, call 1-800-606-NWCR.

What are some positive and negative predictors for successful weight loss/maintenance?

Long-term maintenance of weight loss is the most difficult aspect of treatment. Interventions that provide people with a maintenance program produce better maintenance of weight loss than those without a follow-up program. The expectation of the person, and often the claim of the weight loss programs, is that all excess weight will be lost and kept off. The reality is that weight regain is all too common. Regain is a complex phenomenon and may be facilitated by biological indicators causing a disorder of energy metabolism or by psychological factors such as interpersonal problems leading to dysfunction.

Predictors of Weight Loss Maintenance (185)	
Positive Predictors	**Negative Predictors**
Physical activity	Negative life event
Self-Monitoring	Family dysfunction
Positive coping style	
Continued contact with treatment program	
Normalization of eating	
Reduction of comorbidities	

For most people, the American lifestyle is conducive to obesity and to regain after treatment, given the abundance of food (particularly high-fat foods), huge portion sizes, and limited opportunities for physical activity. For people with a history of overweight or obesity, managing weight becomes a life-long battle. Both the Finnish Diabetes Study (140) and the Diabetes Prevention Program (139) demonstrated that structured and intensive lifestyle-change programs are effective for weight management. The public health community and all health care professionals are challenged to develop effective programs to deal with obesity, the principal public health nutrition problem in the US. LOOK AHEAD is a new multicenter, National Institutes of Health-sponsored research study designed to evaluate the long-term health effects of weight loss in overweight people with type 2 diabetes regarding cardiovascular morbidity and mortality. For more information about LOOK AHEAD, visit http://www.niddk.nih.gov/patient/show/lookahead.htm.

What is the recommended weight loss goal?

The recommended goal for initial weight loss is to reduce body weight by ~10% from baseline. Randomized trials have provided strong and consistent evidence that overweight and obese people in well-designed programs can achieve an average of 7–8% reduction (119,186). A reasonable timeline for a 10% reduction in body weight is 6 months of therapy.

For people who are overweight with body mass indexes in the range of 27–35, a decrease of 300–500 kcal/day will result in weight losses of about 0.5–1 lb/week and a 10% loss in 6 months. For people more severely obese, with body mass indexes >35, deficits of 500–1,000 kcal/day will lead to weight losses of about 1–2 lb/week and a 10% weight loss in 6 months. After 6 months, the rate of weight loss usually declines and weight plateaus because of a lower energy expenditure at the lower weight. Some hypothesize that this weight loss plateau is attributable to compensatory mechanisms to prevent starvation. The role that hormones, such as leptin, gherlin, melacortins, and neuropeptide Y, play in appetite control is a major area of obesity research today.

After 6 months of weight loss treatment, efforts to maintain weight loss should begin. Experience reveals lost weight usually will be regained unless a structured intensive lifestyle change program including medical nutrition therapy, physical activity, and behavior therapy is continued indefinitely.

There is no reason not to continue weight loss treatment if after 6 months the person needs and wants to lose more weight. Continued weight loss generally requires further adjustments of the nutrition and physical activity prescriptions. For people who are unable to achieve significant weight loss, prevention of further weight gain is an important goal; such people can benefit from participation in a structured, intensive lifestyle change program.

What are the benefits of weight loss for people with diabetes?

Obesity is clearly associated with increased morbidity and mortality (119). There is strong evidence that weight loss in overweight and obese individuals reduces risk factors for diabetes and cardiovascular disease. Strong evidence exists that weight loss reduces blood pressure in both overweight hypertensive and nonhypertensive individuals, reduces serum triglycerides and increases high-density lipoprotein cholesterol, and generally produces some reduction in total serum cholesterol and low-density lipoprotein cholesterol. Weight loss reduces blood glucose levels in overweight and obese people with and without diabetes and also reduces blood glucose levels and glycated hemoglobin A1C in some patients with type 2 diabetes. Although there have been no prospective trials to show changes in mortality with weight loss in people who are obese, reductions in risk factors would suggest that development of type 2 diabetes and cardiovascular disease would be reduced with weight loss. The Diabetes Prevention Program demonstrated that weight loss of 7% of initial body weight and 150 min of physical activity/week can prevent diabetes in individuals with impaired glucose tolerance for ~3 years (186).

Who should be considered for bariatric surgery, and what are the primary issues people should consider?

Surgery is one option for weight loss in some people with severe and resistant obesity. According to the National Institutes of Health Consensus Statement for Severe Obesity, people with body mass index >40 and those with body mass index of 35–40 who have high-risk comorbid conditions or significant obesity-related physical conditions that interfere with their lifestyle are candidates for surgery (119). Many obesity experts believe that weight-loss surgery should be reserved for people in whom other methods have failed and who are suffering from the complications of obesity (119). One study suggested that surgery should be considered an early intervention in severely obesity patients with type 2 diabetes (187).

The aim of surgery is to modify the gastrointestinal tract to reduce net food intake. Surgical interventions commonly used include gastroplasty, gastric banding, and gastric bypass. Considerable progress has been made in developing safer and more effective surgical procedures for promoting weight loss. Surgical approaches can result in substantial weight loss of 110 lb to as much as 220 lb over a period of 6 months to 1 year (188).

Compared to other interventions available, surgery has produced the longest period of sustained weight loss. Patients opting for surgical intervention should be followed by a multidisciplinary team (i.e., medical, behavioral, and nutritional professionals). An integrated program should be in place that will provide guidance concerning the necessary eating plan, appropriate physical activity, and behavioral and social support both before and after the surgical procedure. Identification of psychological issues and initiation of healthy eating habits before surgery is strongly recommended.

Assessing both perioperative risk and long-term complications is important and requires assessing the risk/benefit ratio in each case (189). Overeating can cause pouch stretching, band erosion or slippage, and staple rupturing. Because surgical procedures result in some loss of absorptive function, the long-term consequences of potential nutrient deficiencies must be recognized and adequate monitoring performed, particularly with regard to vitamin B12, folate, and iron. Some people may develop gastrointestinal symptoms such as chronic vomiting, "dumping syndrome," or gallstones. Recommended eating plans vary according to individual tolerances. Taking tiny bites of food, chewing food very well, and giving up certain foods must become a way of life to avoid suffering severe stomach pains, vomiting, or diarrhea. Occasionally, people may have postoperative mood changes or their presurgical depression symptoms may not be improved by the achieved weight loss. Thus, rigorous medical monitoring is required postsurgically. Hospital readmissions and reoperations are often necessary. Complications of gastric surgery most commonly include wound infections, intraabdominal abscesses, hernias, pulmonary emboli, nutrient deficiencies, and anemia.

Encourage candidates to

- look for a facility with a team of medical, surgical, psychological, and nutrition experts who can evaluate readiness for the surgery.
- ask about the program's complication rate, including mortality risk. Expect mortality risk to be <0.5%, or <1 in 200.
- make sure there is follow-up care once they are released. Some programs offer support groups and even access to individual counseling. Ideally, there should be life-long follow-up care.
- choose a surgeon who has performed at least 25 obesity operations at a rate of at least two per week.

How can depression affect eating behaviors, and what is the best approach for an obese person who is depressed?

Depression is a common and critically important phenomenon among people with diabetes, affecting 15–20%. The odds of depression are higher in people with diabetes than in those without diabetes (190). Depression in people with diabetes is associated with increased health care use and expenditures. Although equally common in people with type 1 or type 2 diabetes, studies suggest that depression occurs more frequently in women than men. Often unrecognized in the clinical setting, once present, depression will interact negatively with diabetes and the components of diabetes management (191). Depression has been associated with poor glycemic control and diabetes complications. Specifically, depression is associated with obesity and physical inactivity. People who are depressed may be less responsive to appropriate lifestyle interventions in these areas as well (192). They typically consume more high-fat foods and desserts or sweets than people who are not depressed. Depression in combination with alcohol abuse is common; excess drinking can be a symptom of severe clinical depression, or depression may result from prolonged alcohol abuse.

Screening for depression needs to be part of the medical history in people with diabetes and should be evaluated by all health care providers. If depression is suspected, the person with diabetes should be referred for further evaluation and treatment. People with major depression typically experience significant changes in appetite and body weight. These include a weight gain of more than 5% of body weight within a month and a self-reported increase in appetite nearly every day (191). Also, most depression medications are associated with some weight gain. The depressed person may be characterized by feelings of worthlessness or inappropriate guilt, which contribute to patterns of negative thinking with the resulting failure to lose weight. Diminished ability to think or concentrate leads to impaired problem-solving ability that may cripple efforts to control diabetes and/or body weight and potentiate the cycle of negative thinking. Negative thinking itself is a stressor and a factor in worsening of glucose control. When depression is complicated by alcoholism or substance abuse, this further interferes with weight loss. Depression responds well to some lifestyle therapies, particularly physical activity, because physical activity functions as a potent antidepressant. An array of antidepressant medications is available.

Special Populations

OLDER PEOPLE

If an older adult with type 2 diabetes is not using insulin, is there any reason to ask the person to do self-monitoring of blood glucose?

Yes. Older adults with type 2 diabetes should use a blood glucose meter for the same reason as anyone else living with diabetes—to determine how well their treatment regimen is working (193). Glucose monitoring provides feedback so people can see for themselves what changes, especially food choices, are likely to improve their diabetes care.

Through monitoring, older adults may see what extra food from a restaurant meal or late-night snack did to their fasting glucose level. They may discover that sleepiness after dinner may be related to elevated postprandial glucose. If they are hesitant to switch from regular to diet soft drinks, monitoring results can help illustrate the benefit. Blood glucose monitoring results provide factual information on which to base recommendations. They may discover that their glucose levels are high all the time no matter what they do, a clue that medication changes and/or additions are needed. Monitoring provides information with which to problem solve.

Testing frequency can vary greatly depending on the information needed, cost, and patient willingness. As usual, there is no one answer. Vision, dexterity, and hearing may influence which meter is most appropriate. Older adults are perhaps more diverse than any other group, including at what age 'older' begins. Some people are 'older' in function and outlook before age 60, and others remain active and engaged past age 90. Sometimes a family member will do the actual testing, and sometimes (perhaps often) the demands of other medical problems override the benefits of monitoring. However, neither age, type of diabetes, or treatment regimen precludes the benefits of self-monitoring of blood glucose (194).

What happens when an older person does not drink adequate fluids, and what should we recommend?

Age tends to bring increased risk for suboptimal fluid status. Many adults experience reduced thirst, reduced taste sensation, and fewer cues to drink. This can be aggravated by depression, excess alcohol, and living alone or in an institutional setting. Inadequate hydration concentrates glucose and increases risk for hyperosmolar hyperglycemic state (see pages 121–123).

Suggest the following to patients to encourage fluid intake.

■ Restrict food and drink only when absolutely necessary (e.g., presurgery).
■ Set up cues for drinking—keep a glass in the bathroom as a reminder to drink every time they go there, post a sign for themselves, keep a glass by TV, and have a preferred drink available (i.e., buy, mix up, put it in a container that is easy to handle).
■ Find acceptable no-calorie or very low–calorie fluids, especially if they do not care for water alone, such as
  ● Kool Aid or lemonade mixes made with nonnutritive sweetener
  ● Diet V-8 Splash (1 cup = 3 g carbohydrate and 10 calories)
  ● Sugar-free Kool Aid or lemonade or diet V-8 Splash diluted with water to make them less sweet
  ● Lemonade or limeade made by mixing water, nonnutritive sweetener, and lemons or limes
  ● Light fruit juice blends (1/2 cup = 5 g carbohydrate and 20 calories)

- Bottled/sparkling water (some are flavored and calorie free, but the check label)
- Hot or iced tea of various flavors (use caution with some herbals)
- Water with juice, lemon, Kool Aid, clear diet drink, or some combination of these
- Diet carbonated drink sweetened with nonnutritive sweetener
- Coffee, preferably decaffeinated (caffeine is a diuretic)

GESTATIONAL DIABETES

Should I be recommending a maximum amount of carbohydrate and restriction of fruit/fruit juice at breakfast for women with gestational diabetes mellitus (GDM)?

Carbohydrate is restricted at breakfast (or any other time) to the extent necessary to achieve clinical goals. Plasma glucose goals for GDM are <105 mg/dl fasting, <155 mg/dl 1 h after meals, and <130 mg/dl 2 h after meals (195). Carbohydrate is generally less tolerated in the morning due to increased levels of cortisol and growth hormone. Consequently, breakfast is the meal that may require the greatest carbohydrate restriction. A moderate restriction to 30–45 g, or as low as 15 g, is sometimes needed to achieve goals.

However, there is no evidence that women with GDM absorb sugar any differently than others with diabetes. Glucose is the form of carbohydrate most rapidly absorbed. Other monosacharides, fructose and galactose, are primarily stored in the liver as glycogen. Only 50% of the sucrose (table sugar) molecule is glucose, whereas starches are long polymers of 100% glucose. Therefore, most sugars have a lower glucose response than starches. The only reason to avoid juice is that other sources of carbohydrate may be more filling when total carbohydrate is limited to less than preferred intake.

Similarly, doughnuts and sweet rolls are discouraged, not because they contain sugar but because they contain a large amount of carbohydrate (and calories) in a small amount of food with few nutrients. Such treats are okay as long as the overall meal plan supports all the clinical goals for pregnancy: glycemic control and adequate calories and nutrients for appropriate growth and development of the fetus and health of the mother (196).

The level of carbohydrate intolerance varies from one individual to the next. One woman may need to carefully measure and distribute carbohydrate between three meals and two to four snacks to avoid hyperglycemia. Others stimulate hyperglycemia only when they eat >90 g carbohydrate at one meal. Some may tolerate 60 g of some foods but not of others. In addition, insulin resistance and therefore glucose intolerance typically increases as the pregnancy progresses. Food records and self-monitoring of blood glucose provide the information necessary to tailor and adjust carbohydrate distribution to meet glycemic goals throughout the pregnancy without imposing unnecessary restrictions.

Common Concerns/Issues

EATING AWAY FROM HOME

What are the most important skills to teach people for eating meals away from home? When should this information be taught?

In the last few decades, eating meals away from home has gone from being a special occasion to a standard part of our fast-paced lifestyle. Today, according to the National Restaurant Association, the average person eats four meals away from home each week. Eating away from home doesn't just mean going to a restaurant to eat a meal. It can mean using the drive-up window at a fast-food restaurant, eating a hot dog and chips at a convenience store or ball park, or having a slice of pizza in a food court or during an after-work meeting. In addition, restaurant foods are not just eaten away from home. People commonly purchase restaurant meals to eat at home or ready-to-eat meals from the supermarket (e.g., a chicken dinner, deli food, pizza, or Chinese food). Simply stated: food is much more prevalent and accessible than it has ever been.

Unfortunately, the foods that are often available away from home are higher in added sugars, total and saturated fat, cholesterol, and sodium. Whole grains, fruits, and vegetables are often not part of the mix. All of these factors combined make healthy eating particularly difficult for people with diabetes.

As you assess a patient's food intake and habits, ask the following questions:

- How often do you purchase/eat away from home? Daily? Weekly? Monthly?
- Which meals and/or snacks do you most frequently eat away from home?
- What types of restaurants or other food outlets do you frequent?
- What are several of your common orders at various restaurants?
- Are there foods you purchase at restaurants or other outlets and bring home for meals or parts of meals?

Patients' responses will help you gauge when (or if) you teach about restaurant eating, the type of information they need (e.g., skills and information for fast food or fine dining), and how much time to spend on the subject. Be realistic and practical in your approach to this topic (197,198). Allow the types of restaurants and the types of foods to guide the advice you provide. The traditional advice for restaurant eating so often found in basic teaching materials (such as call ahead to find out what the restaurant serves, order with sauce on the side, or order broth as a starter) is not very helpful.

Teaching points about restaurant foods:

- Acknowledge the pitfalls of foods/meals purchased and/or eaten away from home, such as portions, fat content, large servings of meat, and sodium content. Use the meals they typically eat at restaurants to demonstrate the problems.
- Ask them whether they can decrease the number of times per week they eat away from home. For example, are they purchasing a breakfast sandwich on the way to work several days a week? So much of a person's eating style is habits and patterns. Help them understand their habits and patterns, and provide suggestions to help them identify alternatives.
- Help people develop applicable skills such as:
  - how to choose foods with lower fat, saturated fat, cholesterol content, and sodium (if a problem)
  - how to choose restaurants that offer some healthier choices, and supply the names of several
  - strategies and tips to control portions and avoid overeating (see pages 130–132 for portion control tips for eating away from home)
  - practice choosing healthier meals at their favorite restaurants
  - practice estimating the carbohydrate content of restaurant meals from available nutrition information (see next page)

Based on your assessment of the person's knowledge and habits, the topic of eating away from home may lend itself to a discussion of alcohol, managing delayed or irregular meal times, and tips for incorporating sweets in a portion-controlled manner. These issues sometimes come up in relation to restaurant meals more often than in discussions about food intake at home.

What nutrition information is available for restaurant foods today?

The amount of nutrition information available for restaurant foods is greater today than ever before, probably due to consumer demand. However, most exact nutrition information is available from national chain restaurants whose service is so-called "walk up and order." It's easy for anyone to find nutrition information for national hamburger, pizza, sub, and breakfast chains on the companies' web sites or in books or booklets/pamphlets. The booklet/pamphlet of nutrition information from a national chain may or may not be available in individual restaurant locations but some chain restaurants post their nutrition information in a chart on the wall. However, national chain restaurants of the "sit down and order" variety continue to provide minimal nutrition information. Generally, they claim they don't have nutrition information because their menu changes frequently and items are made differently from restaurant to restaurant. Some resources to find nutrition information for restaurant foods are listed below.

Internet

Many of the large chain restaurants have web sites that provide nutrition information. Simply guess at the company's web site address (e.g., www.mcdonalds.com or www.pizzahut.com) or search for it using an Internet search engine such as www.google.com. Another useful web site is www.calorieking.com, which has an extensive listing of restaurant foods, including ethnic foods.

Resources

Borushek A: *The Doctor's Pocket Calorie, Fat and Carbohydrates Counter.* Costa Mesa, CA, Family Health Publications, 2000

Jones DR: *Nutrition in the Fast Lane—The Fast Food Dining Guide.* Indianapolis, IN, Franklin Publishing, 2003

Warshaw HS: *Eat Out, Eat Right.* Chicago, Surrey Books, 2003

Warshaw HS: Fast Food and Restaurant Fare (Column). *Diabetes Forecast* June 2001–May 2003 (Each column reviewed one national restaurant chain, providing tips, sample meals at 3 calorie levels, and nutrition information.)

Warshaw HS: *Guide to Healthy Restaurant Eating.* 2nd ed. Alexandria, VA, American Diabetes Association, 2002

Do you have any suggestions for people who don't have much time or interest in preparing meals?

Meals do not need to be fancy or hot to be nutritious. Replacing fast food or carry-out dinners with a few simple meals at home is likely to provide more nutrients for fewer calories and probably for less money. Food prepared at home is usually a better choice even if it is not the best possibility. For example, a bologna sandwich will be less fat and calories than a cheeseburger and fries. A few ideas to consider are:

- soup and sandwich
- eggs, toast, and fruit
- sandwich or bagel with cheese, plus fruit and/or raw vegetable
- salad bar take-home meal with meat/cheese/egg and light dressing; add carbohydrate with chickpeas, fresh fruit, crackers, or a roll
- peanut butter and banana sandwich
- cottage cheese, fruit, crackers/toast/roll
- crunchy unsweetened cereal with fresh fruit and nuts in light yogurt
- frozen meals/entrees (e.g., Healthy Choice is one brand that is modified for sugar, fat, and sodium) plus fruit/

milk/bread/salad to supplement (the 250- to 350-calorie meals are rarely enough food alone)

■ all-in-one frozen stir-fry dinners

Here are some ideas that make cooking at home easier.

■ Try a combination soup or stew. This is a great way to use leftovers. Combine a source of protein (e.g., leftover meat, chicken from the can, light sausage), starch (e.g., potato, pasta, corn, peas, pinto beans), vegetables (a bag from the freezer will do), water, and something to add flavor (e.g., broth, bullion, light cream soup, dried soup mix, tomato juice/sauce/stewed or gravy mix, and spices). Simmer on low, ideally in a crockpot.

■ Use prepared vegetables such as broccoli and cauliflower from salad bar, mini vegetable trays, and bagged salads.

■ Use a raw vegetable instead of a salad or cooked one, like baby carrots, grape tomatoes, cucumbers, green pepper.

■ Try frozen meatless (grain) burgers cooked in the microwave or on the outside grill.

■ Cook unhusked corn on the cob in the microwave. Allow cooling slightly before husking. There are no dishes to wash, and taste is sealed in.

■ Delegate grilling of lean meat, put potato in the microwave, and pour a bagged salad in a bowl.

HYPOGLYCEMIA/HYPERGLYCEMIA/SICK DAYS

What is the difference between diabetic ketoacidosis (DKA) and hyperosmolar hyperglycemic state (HHS)?

DKA typically occurs in people with type 1 diabetes but may develop in later stages of type 2 diabetes when insulin production is marginal (199, 200). In addition, youth with undiagnosed type 2 diabetes can present in DKA. DKA develops quickly and is often precipitated by missed insulin doses or excess stress hormones. Unfortunately, insulin is too often skipped intentionally as a way to lose weight or perhaps to avoid injections during work or school hours. Infection and illness stimulate stress hormones to the extent that usual doses of injected insulin do not keep pace with the increased glucose production by the liver. Stress from injury, depression, and anxiety may do the same. Increased insulin needs during growth spurts and expired insulin are additional reasons. Symptoms of DKA may include nausea, vomiting, stomach pain, thirst, and fruity breath.

The primary cause of DKA is profound insulin deficiency, leading to ketosis, osmotic diuresis, and electrolyte imbalances. Blood pH will be elevated, and serum glucose typically ranges from 250 to 600 mg/dl. DKA is treated with insulin, fluids (~3–5 oz/h), and electrolytes based on laboratory results. Supplemental potassium is usually necessary.

Prevention for DKA lies primarily in education. Patients may avoid serious complications if they know to take insulin even when eating little or nothing (due to stress hormones causing glucose production by liver) and to drink fluids regularly (due to extra losses from fever, diarrhea, or glycosuria). Because glucose levels are much less predictable during illness, more frequent monitoring of blood glucose and testing for ketones provide the information needed to act to prevent DKA. Probe reasons for omitted insulin, and refer the patient for counseling if appropriate (201).

HHS is much rarer than DKA and typically occurs in undiagnosed or elderly people with type 2 diabetes whether or not they are taking oral diabetes medications. HHS develops slowly over several days or weeks and is most common in hospitalized or nursing home patients. An impaired thirst mechanism, common in aging adults, may exacerbate fluid losses from diarrhea, fever, diuretics or dialysis, and cause shortness of breath and mental changes.

The primary cause of HHS is profound dehydration accompanied by increased plasma osmolality. Ketone levels are not elevated, but serum glucose may range from 600 to 2,000 mg/dl. Careful rehydration is essential; insulin may or may not be required. The extreme glucose elevation is due to gross concentration of glucose from inadequate fluids. Excess food or inadequate insulin may worsen the event.

Symptoms of HHS are less noticeable because they develop slowly. Typical symptoms are elevated blood glucose levels rising over several days and polyuria for several days or even weeks. Patients may exhibit neurological changes similar to those following a stroke.

Prevention for HHS is adequate hydration, usually overseen by someone beside the patient. Educate and support family members or caretakers who oversee fluid intake for those at risk. More often, the hospital or nursing home staff is responsible for providing and monitoring hydration status.

Resources

American Association of Diabetes Educators: *A CORE Curriculum for Diabetes Educators. Diabetes and Complications.* 5th ed. Franz M, Ed. Chicago, American Association of Diabetes Educators, 2001

American Diabetes Association: *Managing Diabetic Hypoglycemia* (Videocassette). Alexandria, VA, American Diabetes Association, 2000 (Provides patient education on hypoglycemia and DKA.)

How should sick days be managed in people with diabetes?

Not all sick days affect food intake or timing of medication. On sick days during which people can maintain their usual food intake and medication schedule, they should do so. But colds, fever, flu, vomiting, and diarrhea—all common illnesses—can cause special problems for people with diabetes. If not handled appropriately, these types of short-term illness in people using insulin or insulin secretogogues can quickly result in elevated blood glucose levels. During illness, stress hormones increase, leading to the need for more insulin than usual. In fact, stress hormones raise blood glucose levels higher than eating does. Therefore, individuals must take their insulin or insulin secretogogue even if they are eating less than normal due to nausea or vomiting.

During illness individuals must test their blood glucose levels and test their blood or urine for ketones. If glucose is >250 mg/dl, it is especially important to test for ketones. The combination of elevated blood glucose and moderate-to-large ketones signals the need for additional insulin. Teach patients to call their health care provider if this happens.

Patients also must drink adequate amounts of fluid and eat or drink some form of carbohydrate, especially if their blood glucose is <100 mg/dl (202). To prevent dehydration, a large glass of calorie-free liquid (e.g., water, diet soft drinks, tea) should be ingested every hour. A patient who feels nauseated or is vomiting should take small sips of liquid (e.g., 1–2 Tbsp every 15–30 min). Replacement fluids containing sodium, such as broth or sports drinks, are also helpful. To prevent starvation ketosis (i.e., ketones from the breakdown of fat caused by lack of glucose available for energy), ~150–200 g carbohydrate/day are needed (124). Individuals should eat 45–50 g carbohydrate every 3–4 h. If regular food is not tolerated, liquid or soft carbohydrate foods, such as regular (not diet) soft drinks, juices, soups, and ice cream can be eaten.

Instruct patients to call their health care provider immediately if they have any of the following symptoms:

■ They are vomiting and haven't been able to keep any liquids or carbohydrate down for >3–4 h.

- They test positive for ketones in urine or blood.
- They begin to breathe rapidly or become drowsy. If they lose consciousness, someone must immediately call for assistance.

Insulin should never be omitted. Supplementary insulin may also be needed. When the illness is over, patients can return to their regular food/meal plan and insulin schedule. If they need help with continued insulin adjustments, instruct them to call or visit their health care provider.

What do people with diabetes need to understand about managing hypoglycemia?

First, people with diabetes need to learn about their personal risk for hypoglycemia. Many people believe that they are at risk for hypoglycemia simply because they have diabetes. Correct that notion, and advise that the risk of hypoglycemia is due to the chosen medication regimen, not simply the diagnosis of diabetes. Hypoglycemia is not a risk when medications such as insulin sensitizers are used as the only blood glucose–lowering medication. Hypoglycemia is a risk for people who take any type(s) of insulin and/or insulin secretegogues, especially if their medication isn't synchronized with their current eating pattern.

Clinicians and people with type 2 diabetes facing the need to go on insulin often cite hypoglycemia as an adverse effect of insulin therapy and one that precludes its use. However, studies do not support this notion; rates of severe hypoglycemia are quite low in type 2 diabetes patients (203). The Kumamoto study demonstrated only mild hypoglycemic reactions and similar rates of hypoglycemia in both the tight control and conventional groups (204). The United Kingdom Prospective Diabetes Study found that major hypoglycemic episodes were higher for patients on insulin (2.3%) than for patients on any other intensive or conventional therapy (<1%) (126). The rate of any hypoglycemic episode was 36.5% with insulin treatment, compared to 18%, 11%, and 1% with the sulfonylureas glibenclamide and chlorpropamide and nutrition monotherapy, respectively. In a secondary analysis of obese patients on intensive glycemic control, the rate of major hypoglycemic events per year for intensive insulin treatment was 2.5% vs. <1% for other treatments.

To determine what a person needs to learn about hypoglycemia, assess

- whether they are at risk for hypoglycemia
- whether they currently have occasional hypoglycemia or a pattern of hypoglycemia. If so, why? Determine whether a change in an aspect of management (e.g., medications, food, timing of activity) would decrease the likelihood of hypoglycemia
- whether they have the knowledge to detect hypoglycemia symptoms and treat various degrees of hypoglycemia

Teach people at risk for hypoglycemia

- about their potential for hypoglycemia due to their blood glucose–lowering medication
- the symptoms of early and late hypoglycemia
- how to prevent hypoglycemia between meals and during the night
- proper treatment of hypoglycemia between meals, during and after physical activity, and during the night
- about sources of glucose/carbohydrate that are easy to carry and have accessible whenever and wherever
- about the need to have sources of glucose/carbohydrate available and accessible at all times
- strategies for not overtreating hypoglycemia
- locations to keep glucose/carbohydrate (e.g., glove compartment; purse, pocket, or knapsack; desk or locker; night table)

- about the importance of training others to manage/treat an unconscious hypoglycemic episode (e.g., using glucagons and/or calling 911)

Once these concepts about hypoglycemia are learned, encourage patients to tailor their treatment of hypoglycemia based on their experiences. They should learn about their own early and late symptoms; how much carbohydrate they need to treat a mild, moderate, and severe episode of hypoglycemia with blood glucose testing results; what sources of glucose/carbohydrate work best; and the best locations to have various treatments.

If a person has any degree of hypoglycemia unawareness, additional education is needed. It is especially important that the patient teach others about the actions to be taken when severe hypoglycemia develops because early signs were absent. Advice that the patient may have received early in his or her diabetes education may need to be revised; blood glucose goals may need to be higher, and he or she may need to set a higher blood glucose level at which to treat a reaction.

What is the best treatment for hypoglycemia?

Although any form of carbohydrate that contains glucose can be used for treatment, 100% glucose is preferred. Initial responses to treatment with 15–20 g carbohydrate will be seen in ~10–20 min; however, glucose levels need to be evaluated again in ~60 min, as additional treatment may be needed. Typically 15 g carbohydrate will raise glucose levels ~40–50 mg/dl, which would return glucose concentrations to a typical target range from 50 mg/dl. Lower glucose levels may require 20–30 g carbohydrate. Regardless of the guidelines, individuals respond differently, and glucose levels must be monitored.

These guidelines were developed from a study of the treatment of insulin-induced hypoglycemia in which

10 g oral glucose raised plasma glucose levels from 60 to 97 mg/dl over 30 min, with the levels starting to fall after 60 min (205). When the amount was doubled (20 g), plasma glucose levels increased from 58 to 122 mg/dl over 45 min, with the levels again starting to fall after 60 min. Glucose, therefore, is an effective but temporary treatment for hypoglycemia.

Two studies were conducted to determine the preferred treatment of hypoglycemia. In one, subjects with type 1 diabetes and blood glucose levels of 55 mg/dl were treated with 20 g carbohydrate as milk, orange juice, or glucose (206). The response to milk or orange juice (20 g) was approximately half the response of glucose (20 g), which reached a peak level of 110 mg/dl at 40 min.

In the second study, hypoglycemia was treated with 15 g carbohydrate from glucose, sucrose, corn syrup, glucose gel, or orange juice. The response to glucose, sucrose, or corn syrup began between 2 and 3 min and at 10 min was similar, with symptoms being alleviated in ~15 min; however, at 10 min, there was no response to glucose gel or orange juice (after 10 min glucose levels did begin to increase but never reached the peak effect of glucose, sucrose, or corn syrup) (207). This study illustrates that there are no "fast-acting" carbohydrates for the treatment of hypoglycemia and that all carbohydrates eventually raise blood glucose levels.

Furthermore, there appears to be no advantage of liquid over solid carbohydrate sources in the treatment of hypoglycemia, as is often suggested to person with diabetes. The rate of gastric emptying of both liquids and solids was increased to ~15 min during hypoglycemia compared to 40 min during normoglycemia (208). Thus, the emptying rates for the solid and liquid tests were similar.

Adding protein or fat to treatment only adds unnecessary and often unwanted calories. In a study of insulin-induced hypoglycemia, treatments with 15 g carbohydrate or 15 g carbohydrate plus 15 g protein were compared

(209). Neither the posttreatment glucose peak nor the subsequent rate of fall in glucose differed. Foods high in fat may also delay the peak glucose response.

Not to be forgotten are convenience and acceptable taste. The reason foods that have been traditionally recommended, such as regular soft drinks, fruit juice, honey, and LifeSavers, remain good choices are not because they treat hypoglycemia better than other carbohydrates but because they are convenient, readily available, easily and quickly consumed, don't spoil, and have an enjoyable taste.

It is common for patients to overtreat hypoglycemia. Teach them to wait and recheck glucose levels after 15 min to prevent hyperglycemia, instead of eating until symptoms disappear. Help patients understand that incorporating sweets into their planned meals or snacks instead of using them as free foods during hypoglycemia helps prevent hyperglycemia.

What can people with diabetes do to manage their blood glucose levels on days when the timing of food intake is inconsistent?

Teach people with diabetes to eat a consistent amount of carbohydrate at similar times of the day and from day to day to help keep their blood glucose in target range. Those who take insulin or an insulin secretegogue need to know that skipping or delaying meals or not eating sufficient carbohydrate at a meal, without making a matching change in medication, puts them at risk for hypoglycemia.

However, it is unrealistic due to the hectic and varied pace of life today to suggest that people will be able to do this day after day. Assess whether the person's current medication regimen is providing the level of flexibility their lifestyle requires. If not, explore a more flexible medication plan, with the goal of fitting the person's lifestyle into a diabetes plan, not the opposite.

With that said, the most important skill to teach is how to problem solve in the various situations of daily life, such as delayed or missed meals, extended or unexpected activity, or traveling across time zones. To cope with such situations, people need to have portable, nonperishable, yet healthy snacks always available, such as dried or fresh fruit, pretzels, popcorn, crackers, dry cereal, and the like. Depending on the type of medication a person takes, they may be encouraged to omit, take more or less, or change the timing of one or more medications for certain situations.

PORTION CONTROL

Why is portion control important, and what are the concepts and skills to convey to patients about it?

One culprit of our current epidemic of obesity, pre-diabetes, and type 2 diabetes is that the portions of foods and beverages served both in the home and at restaurants have increased during the last two decades (210,211). The greatest increase in portions has been in fast-food restaurants and the home (210). People are encouraged to overeat on a regular basis. Therefore, teaching the concepts and strategies of portion control is critical.

First, suggest that patients eat 25% less than their current intake. With this strategy, they can continue to eat and enjoy the foods they are used to. To do this, they need to learn to judge portion sizes. Provide guidelines of reasonable portions for various types and preparations of foods and a handout with "handy" hand guides (see page 132) and common objects. Encourage the use of measuring equipment when the person eats at home. Determine whether they have a set of measuring cups and spoons as well as a food scale. A resource for food scales beyond the usual postage scale is The Diabetes Mall at www.diabetes net.com. Encourage people to keep their measuring equipment out on a counter where it is easy to see and use. Realistically, most people do not continue to weigh and measure foods daily after the initial learning period. Once a person has educated him- or herself about portions, encourage the use of measuring equipment once a week or once a month to maintain visual accuracy, which is vital to estimating portions of restaurant foods.

Teaching points for practicing portion control for eating at home:

- Advise people to eat just the serving size of foods given in Nutrition Facts on food labels.
- When purchasing produce—fruits, vegetables, and starches—buy the smallest ones. Look for small apples, bananas, and potatoes.
- Use smaller plates, such as a lunch-size plate versus a dinner plate. Large dinner plates promote overfilling the plate and then overeating.
- Purchase and prepare the amount of food needed for meals serving reasonable portions. Do not prepare too much food unless you plan on leftovers. If you plan on leftovers, put the extra food away before serving.
- Don't serve family style (i.e., placing bowls, pots, or casserole pans on the table). This makes overeating too easy because more food is in front of people and just an arm's reach away. If people want seconds, at least make them get up from the table.
- If the habit of eating seconds is difficult to break, consider splitting the portions into two servings—firsts and seconds.
- Weighing and measuring foods at home trains the eyes to estimate portions when eating restaurant foods.

Teaching points for practicing portion control for eating restaurant meals (197,198):

- Do not order menu items with portion descriptors such as giant, grande, supreme, extra large, jumbo, double, triple, double-decker, king size, and super—unless you split them. Order menu items that mean small such as junior, single, queen, petite, kiddie, and regular.

- Do not up-size portions or be taken in by deals or bargains that promote overeating.
- Avoid all-you-can-eat restaurants or buffets. They simply encourage overeating.
- Be creative with menus. Don't automatically order a main course. Opt for a soup and salad, or appetizer and soup, or soup and appetizer. Order a half portion or eat family style—share a few menu items.
- Split, share, and mix and match menu items to eat in desirable portions.
- Use the portion-estimating abilities developed from weighing and measuring foods at home.
- If the portion served will be too large, ask for a take-home container to be brought when the meal is served. Put away the extras before starting the meal.

Use these "handy" hand guides to get a feel for reasonable portions. They are always with you—at home or out.

Thumb tip = 1 tsp
    Example: 1 tsp mayonnaise or margarine
Thumb or ping pong ball = 1 oz or 2 Tbsp
    Example: 1 oz cheese or meat
Palm or deck of cards = 3 oz
    Example: 3 oz cooked meat (with no bone)
Tight fist, tennis ball, bar of soap, or ice cream
    scoop = 1/2 cup
    Example: 1 serving of cooked cereal or canned fruit
Handful = 1 cup

NUTRITION LABEL

What are the most important elements of and concepts to teach about the food label?

Food labels include information about the food (e.g., name and address of manufacturer, weight in grams and ounces), possibly a nutrition (e.g., no sugar added, low-fat, reduced calorie) and/or health (e.g., may decrease the risk of cancer or heart disease) claim, a Nutrition Facts panel, and a list of ingredients. Food labels provide the educator with excellent teaching tools because they are easy to obtain, inexpensive, and familiar to the patient. Using these in teaching helps the patient when they shop for food.

Begin by orienting a person to the elements of the food label. Note the Nutrition Facts, the ingredients, and the location and wording of possible nutrition and/or health claims. Explain that the nutrients on the Nutrition Facts are provided by one serving of the food. Teach clients to use the food label to estimate the amount of carbohydrate (or other nutrient of concern) that is in one serving of the food. If they eat more or less than one serving, they will need to calculate the amount of carbohydrate (or other nutrient of concern) in the portion they will actually eat. Have sample labels available for teaching from common single foods, such as packaged fruits, vegetables, and cereals as well as combination foods, such as frozen pizza or a frozen entrée.

People, especially those newly diagnosed with diabetes or those with insufficient education, will commonly focus their attention in the supermarket on the amount of sugars indicated on the food label. Teach them to look at the total carbohydrate as an indicator of how the product may affect their blood glucose, for three reasons:

- The sugars are counted within the total carbohydrates. Note how sugar and dietary fiber are indented and in lighter print than the total carbohydrates.
- People assume that the sugars in a food are simply the added sugars. In fact, the sugars are defined by Food and Drug Administration as all the mono- and disaccharides. This includes both the naturally occurring sugars, such as lactose in milk and fructose in fruit, and the added sugars, such as high-fructose corn syrup, sugar, dextrose, or brown sugar.

■ The main focus should be on the amount of total carbohydrate they consume and the total carbohydrate in a
food product, rather than the source or type of carbohydrate. Understand that carbohydrates are starches, sugars, and dietary fibers.

Drawing attention to the serving sizes of various products is a good way to teach people about the definition of a
reasonable portion. Today's serving sizes on food labels
are called reference servings and are defined and regulated
by Food and Drug Administration. This makes servings
consistent between products and makes comparisons
between products easier. Serving sizes in Nutrition Facts
must be provided in both grams and in common household measures. A serving size might read 30 g (1 oz) or 6
crackers or 1/2 cup. Encourage people to use the household measures because they are most understandable. Be
sure people understand the gram weight of a food is different from the grams of carbohydrate (or other nutrients) it
contains.

People should understand that the ingredients are listed
in descending order of quantity based on weight. They can
be encouraged to use the ingredient list to look for a particular ingredient to include or exclude from their diet. For
example, to limit *trans* fats, encourage people to limit partially hydrogenated fats and oils in the ingredient list.
Knowing the common names of saturated fats, such as
coconut or palm kernel oil; polyols, such as sorbitol, mannitol, or polydextrose; or no-calorie sweeteners, such as
aspartame or sucralose, can help people identify ingredients to include or exclude from their diet.

Food labels can help teach people about nutrition and
health claims. For people with diabetes, it is most important that they understand the meaning of the nutrition
claims "sugar-free" and "no sugar added." Compare the

Nutrition Facts

Serving Size 1 cup (228g)
Servings Per Container 2

Amount Per Serving

Calories 260   Calories from Fat 120

	% Daily Value*
Total Fat 13g	**20%**
Saturated Fat 5g	**25%**
Cholesterol 30mg	**10%**
Sodium 660mg	**28%**
Total Carbohydrate 31g	**10%**
Dietary Fiber 0g	**0%**
Sugars 5g	
Protein 5g	

Vitamin A 4%	•	Vitamin C 2%
Calcium 15%	•	Iron 4%

* Percent Daily Values are based on a 2,000 calorie diet. Your daily values may be higher or lower depending on your calorie needs:

	Calories:	2,000	2,500
Total Fat	Less than	65g	80g
Sat Fat	Less than	20g	25g
Cholesterol	Less than	300mg	300mg
Sodium	Less than	2,400mg	2,400mg
Total Carbohydrate		300g	375g
Dietary Fiber		25g	30g

Calories per gram:
Fat 9 • Carbohydrate 4 • Protein 4

labels from a regular ice cream and a sugar-free ice cream to illustrate the minimal calorie and carbohydrate reduction afforded by the sugar-free ice cream. Help them understand that sugar-free doesn't necessarily mean calorie or carbohydrate free. It's also important to teach that products that are low fat or fat free may contain so-called carbohydrate-based fat replacers, such as polyols or starches, that may lower the fat content but in turn raise the carbohydrate content (see pages 17–19).

Resources

The FDA is the US government agency that has main jurisdiction over the Nutrition Facts label. Access information about food labeling on the FDA web site at www.cfsan.fda. gov/label.html
Reading Food Labels: A Handbook for People with Diabetes (Pamphlet). Alexandria, VA, American Diabetes Association, and Dallas, TX, American Heart Association, 2002

SNACKING

Should people with diabetes be encouraged or discouraged to snack between meals to help control their blood glucose levels?

An eating plan for people with diabetes should no longer automatically include snacks. The rationale for including snacks in years past was to prevent hypoglycemia due to diabetes medications. People are at less risk of hypoglycemia due to diabetes medications today because of newer oral medications, some of which don't cause hypoglycemia, and newer insulins, both rapid acting and longer acting. In addition, with the advent of blood glucose monitoring, people are able to know their blood glucose level at any time and treat it accordingly.

It is well known that decreasing calorie intake to promote weight loss or maintenance is an effective approach to treating type 2 diabetes. One-day studies in people with type 2 diabetes reported that spreading food (same total number of calories) throughout the day in multiple small meals was beneficial in reducing average blood glucose and insulin levels throughout the day. (212,213) One study showed a slight reduction in triglycerides (212). However, when studied in the long term (over several days), food frequency—either three meals or small meals and snacks which were isocaloric—was not associated with long-term differences in glucose, lipids, and insulin responses (214,164). Omitting snacks may help an overweight person adhere more closely to a calorie-intake goal because they are minimizing the potential to overeat several times a day. However, the people who want to lose or maintain weight may find that eating several small meals spaced regularly through the day helps them be less hungry and likely to overeat at mealtimes. No studies to date have been conducted to demonstrate that meal eating vs. multiple snacks is more beneficial for calorie reduction and/or weight loss.

Also, the physiologic defect early in the course of type 2 diabetes is a delayed and/or diminished first-phase insulin release. Due to a slower release of insulin, it can take 4–5 hours after food intake to normalize blood glucose levels. Frequent snacking between meals would not allow sufficient time to achieve normal blood glucose levels. However, if a person can control their calorie intake more successfully with five or six small meals a day, their blood glucose excursions, each time they eat, might be diminished.

Therefore, the inclusion or exclusion of snacks for people with diabetes should depend solely on their personal desire to snack and whether they are at a phase of life, such as a toddler or preschooler, when snacks are necessary. If a person regularly includes snacks, ask about their rationale for doing so. Some people with diabetes, their care providers, and family members still have the misconception that people with diabetes, regardless of their medication regimen, must eat every few hours. Advise them that this is no longer true due to medication advancements that lower the risk of hypoglycemia. Discuss when the patient takes their medication(s). It is possible that the improper and/or irregular timing of medication could be causing hypoglycemia. Work with each patient to find an eating plan—inclusive or exclusive of snacks—that works best for their lifestyle and food habits.

When people with diabetes use regimens that combine long-acting basal and rapid-acting mealtime insulins, snacking is not necessary to keep blood glucose within target range or prevent hypoglycemia. If someone is on a less-flexible insulin regimen (i.e., two daily insulin injections of NPH and regular insulin), inform them about the advantages of newer regimens that match carbohydrate intake to insulin dose and determine their interest in a change. If they want to change, be their advocate to help them make this change.

With all these factors in mind, the bottom line is that whether a person does or doesn't snack and the number of snacks they eat each day should be based solely on individual preferences. Snacks should only be included if they are desired by the person, necessary to control blood glucose during activity, or physiologically or nutritionally necessary, such as in infants and small children.

Does protein need to be included in snacks for people using insulin?

No. Individuals with diabetes have traditionally been taught to have a food source of protein before bedtime or to include protein with other snacks or even before exercise. But consider the logic of recommending the addition of 1–2 oz protein to bedtime snacks to prevent overnight hypoglycemia. Even if 50% of the protein was converted to glucose and entered the circulation, this would only be 3.5–7 g glucose. However, it is unlikely that any of the glucose from protein enters the general circulation (see pages 25–27). Even if it did, it is unlikely that this amount of glucose would have much effect on increasing blood glucose levels and preventing hypoglycemia. Therefore, it is doubtful that adding protein to a snack offers any benefit.

A study of bedtime snacks reported that composition of the bedtime snack had minimal effect on glucose levels overnight (215). More important, the need for a snack depended on the glucose level at snack time. No snack was necessary if glucose was >180 mg/dl and at lower levels of glucose, any type of snack could be advised. Unfortunately, the study did not compare a carbohydrate snack alone to a carbohydrate plus protein snack.

To prevent overnight hypoglycemia in insulin users, the following approaches can be tried, although it is unknown which is most helpful: adjusting insulin doses appropriately, ingesting carbohydrate alone, or adding protein to the carbohydrate snack. Perhaps the only reason to even consider adding protein to the snack would be if individuals were still hungry after eating a snack with foods containing carbohydrate. Then, adding extra protein might be better than adding extra carbohydrate.

Prevention of Diabetes

RESOURCES

What important messages have been learned from the Diabetes Prevention Program (DPP)?

The DPP provided clear and strong evidence that both medication and lifestyle interventions can delay or prevent progression from impaired glucose tolerance to type 2 diabetes (186). The timing of this news could not be better, given that experts agree the US is in the midst of an epidemic of obesity and type 2 diabetes (216).

The DPP demonstrated that, compared to the placebo intervention, the intensive lifestyle intervention reduced the incidence of type 2 diabetes by 58% and the metformin intervention reduced the incidence of type 2 diabetes by 31% over 2.8 years. The DPP study population was ethnically diverse, with 45% of participants from minority groups at high risk to develop diabetes. The goal for the lifestyle intervention group was to lose at least 7% of their body weight and increase physical activity to at least 150 min per week. The intensive lifestyle group achieved a 7% weight loss after 1 year of intervention and maintained a 5% weight loss at 3 years (217).

The DPP lifestyle protocol provides a model to demonstrate how lifestyle change to promote modest weight loss and increase physical activity is effective. In the DPP, 50%

of participants reached their weight loss goal, and 74% reached their exercise goal (218). Given the general pessimism surrounding the effectiveness of weight loss interventions, this is powerful and hopeful news. Many of these strategies could be easily incorporated into a clinical practice setting at low cost. Key aspects of the DPP lifestyle protocol included (218):

- continuous focus on clearly defined weight loss and physical activity goals and individual tailoring of treatment for both aspects
- individual counseling focused on fat gram and calorie counting, self-monitoring of blood glucose, behavioral strategies, and physical activity goals
- individual case managers or "lifestyle coaches," with 16 sessions in the first 24 weeks and then at least monthly sessions
- supervised physical activity sessions at least twice weekly
- flexible maintenance programs with motivation campaigns and restart opportunities
- individual "toolbox" strategies, including telephone reminders, contracting, a buddy system, meal replacements, structured menus, gym memberships, and more
- materials/strategies addressing the needs of an ethnically diverse population
- extensive local and national network of training, feedback, and clinical support

The DPP also added support to the growing evidence that meal replacement is a viable approach to the treatment of obesity and should be added to our list of meal planning options (219). Meal replacement involves using formula shakes or bars or prepackaged meals to control portions and simplify food decisions. Typically, formula drinks or bars are used to replace two meals and one snack daily to achieve weight loss and to replace one meal per day for weight maintenance.

What tips can I offer parents to prevent obesity in their children?

Although schools have allowed soda machines on their property to help close budget gaps and now offer brand-name fast foods in the lunchroom, the burden of responsibility to stem the tide of obesity in children lies in the hands of parents. Parents control the grocery shopping for the home and create the family's definition of a meal. Despite the fact that many parents believe they are powerless, parents can and must set rules for what is eaten in the house and when.

Some tips for parents to fight the obesity epidemic in children are (220–222):

- Start cultivating taste buds and eating habits as early as possible. Offer a variety of foods, including vegetables as the first course, when the child is most hungry.
- Be a good role model. You can't expect your children to have good eating habits if you don't have them yourself.
- Don't cook separately for the kids—offer the same foods to the entire family.
- Get the children involved in food preparation. They'll eat more of foods they help prepare.
- Make changes slowly. Pick one habit you want to change per month—e.g., instead of dessert, serve fruit.
- Make sure your children eat breakfast. Make it easy for them to prepare on their own—have whole-grain cereals, fresh fruit, and low-fat milks (including chocolate, if necessary) available.
- Control portions; think in terms of cups and half cups. Serve ice cream in small bowls, not cereal bowls.
- When eating out, never ever "supersize." Think small. Order a small hamburger and small French fries. Use the kid's meals—the portions are right for kids. Order low-fat milk instead of soda or shakes.

- When eating out in sit down restaurants, avoid the kid's menu. The choices are generally not very healthy and they are limited. Teach children how to order from the menu creatively to get smaller portions and/or to split orders or share menu items.
- Don't buy it—chips, soda, doughnuts, candy, etc. Remember, if you buy it, you eat it.
- Stock the house with healthy foods the children like. Put fruits and vegetables in clear sight. Make it "grab and go" as much as possible.
- If you buy soda, avoid large bottles and offer cans.
- Limit the locations for eating to the kitchen and dining room. Avoid bedrooms and eating food in front of the TV. This may also help reduce TV time.
- Make children ask for snacks—parents have more control that way.
- Eat as a family when possible.
- Have set meal times.
- No TV during family meals.
- Put vegetables on their plates. Try one bite for every year of age.
- Don't make treats forbidden. Less available, yes— but not completely banned or you could foster an obsession.
- Monitor frequency of fast-food consumption.
- Avoid overreliance on snack foods bought in bulk at warehouse-style markets.
- Limit TV/computer time.
- Be a role model for an active lifestyle.
- Avoid nagging child to eat more or less of particular food(s).

According to the Centers for Disease Control and the National Center for Health Statistics, in 1999–2000, the prevalence of overweight was 15.5% among 12- to 19-year-olds, 15.3% among 6- to 11-year-olds, and 10.4%

among preschoolers ages 2–5 years, compared with 10.55%, 11.3%, and 7.2%, respectively in 1988–1994 (223). Overweight adolescents have a 70% chance of becoming overweight or obese adults. Type 2 diabetes is being diagnosed in teens and preteens at an alarming rate.

The health consequences of these staggering figures are very serious and include:

- high blood pressure and cardiovascular disease
- type 2 diabetes, formerly a disease of adults
- liver disease
- breathing disorders and sleep apnea
- back pains
- elevated cholesterol
- hip and knee strain
- poor nutrition, especially calcium, vitamins, and fiber, despite being overfed
- depression, low self-esteem, and lack of self-confidence
- chronic health problems that shouldn't happen for decades

Red flags to parents that their child is in danger for serious weight issues are:

- obsession with food—thinking of food as an activity rather than a necessity
- returning to the kitchen repeatedly, after already having eaten
- hoarding or hiding food
- being embarrassed about food habits

The Action for Health Kids Initiative, a nonprofit foundation, has been launched in 51 states and territories to make the fight of healthier school environments a priority at the state and local level. Additional information is available at: www.actionforhealthykids.org and www. childrenshealthfund.org.

Resources

DIETITIAN ACCESS/REFERRAL

How can I help people with diabetes access the services of a dietitian with expertise in diabetes management?

Numerous research studies, such as the MNT effectiveness trials (4,5,224), Diabetes Prevention Program, Finnish prevention trial (139,140), and others (14), show that the services of dietitians with expertise in diabetes management or health care providers trained to coach people in behavior change should be used to provide initial and consistent ongoing education and support. The best way to help a person with diabetes access these services and to reinforce their ability to produce positive outcomes is to provide a written referral to a specific dietitian, diabetes educator, or diabetes education program. Many health care plans require this type of referral.

Because of both state and Federal laws that have been passed during the last two decades, it is more likely now that diabetes self-management training (DSMT) and/or MNT services will be covered (225). This is true for Medicare beneficiaries with Part B coverage and for many people who have private health plans (226–229). Encourage people to call their health plan using the toll-free number on their card to determine their coverage for these services. However, caution patients not to use the words "diabetes education" to describe the service. Unfortunately, health plans don't usually cover education. Instead, patients should describe DSMT and MNT as services that their primary care practitioner has referred them to as a part of their diabetes care. Health plans are more likely to say yes if the service is described as "diabetes care" or "diabetes management."

Refer people to a diabetes education program. At such programs, especially programs that have achieved Recognition in the American Diabetes Association's Education Recognition Program, they will have access to diabetes educators from different disciplines, such as nursing, dietetics, and possibly pharmacy and psychology. Dietitians who work in a diabetes education program are likely to have a special interest and training in diabetes. An additional advantage of referring people to Recognized education programs is that, to date, only programs that have achieved Recognition can seek reimbursement from Medicare. Also, some health plans only cover diabetes education provided by a Recognized program. To find a Recognized program, call 1-800-DIABETES (1-800-342-2383) or visit the American Diabetes Association's web site at http://diabetes.org/education/eduprogram.asp. Make contact with programs in your area and work out specific arrangements for referring your patients.

Resource

Warshaw HS, Daly A: Do you have a dietitian on your team? *Diabetes Forecast* 53:85–88, 2000

How can I reinforce the importance of consistently working with a dietitian with expertise in diabetes?

First, provide a written referral to a diabetes education program. Point out that as part of the diabetes education program, they will be able to work with a dietitian who has expertise in diabetes. Choose a dietitian and/or diabetes education program that is both convenient and with which you/your practice works with regularly. Your written referral is tangible evidence to the patient of your belief in the value of this service to their diabetes care. It is also likely that they will need the written referral if their health plan covers the service (see above).

During follow-up appointments, determine whether the person with diabetes has pursued MNT and/or diabetes education. Find out whether the person has followed through with the diabetes education component of their care. If yes, ask about the experience and the goals they have set for lifestyle changes. If they have not pursued diabetes education, ask why not and about the obstacles to this goal. Again reinforce the benefits of these services in helping them achieve positive outcomes. Subtle messages that you provide about the value and importance of diabetes education can encourage a patient to use these services as a component of their diabetes care.

Health care provider (referral source) responsibilities:

- Refer patient to dietitian for MNT
- Provide referral data: diabetes treatment regimen; laboratory values for glycated hemoglobin A1C, glucose values, cholesterol fractionations, blood pressure, and microalbumin; physician (or team) goals for patient care; medical history; medications that affect nutrition therapy; clearance for exercise
- Communicate patient medical treatment goals to patient
- Based on the outcomes of the nutrition intervention, adjust medications if needed
- Reinforce nutrition self-management education

Dietitian responsibilities (230):

- Obtain referral data and treatment goals before the initial nutrition intervention
- Obtain and assess records about food, exercise, self-monitoring of blood glucose, and psychosocial and economic issues
- Evaluate patient's knowledge, skill level, and readiness to learn
- Identify patient's goals
- Determine and implement an appropriate nutrition prescription
- Provide education on food/meal planning and self-management using appropriate teaching tools
- Evaluate the effectiveness of MNT on medical outcomes, and adjust MNT as needed
- Make recommendations to the physician (or other referral source) based on the outcomes of the nutrition interventions

- Communicate progress/outcomes to all team members
- Plan for follow-up and ongoing MNT and self-management education

What information does a dietitian need to assess someone's dietary needs and make appropriate recommendations?

Meal planning is inter-related to exercise and medication treatments for diabetes. Diabetes dietitians assess nutrition related to hypertension, cardiovascular disease, and obesity as well as renal disease, bone health, and other conditions affected by food choices. People with diabetes are often confused when they have received dissimilar nutritional advice for their heart and blood pressure (and wonder if there will be anything left to eat after a visit to the dietitian who specializes in diabetes care).

To integrate diabetes nutrition recommendations into those for the person's overall health, dietitians require information from the patient's medical record. Otherwise they risk providing nutrition recommendations that are more restrictive than necessary to reach goals.

If the dietitian doesn't have access to the medical record itself, use the following list of helpful information and resources to create referral forms. Practicality may require limiting referral data to the most essential information that is not reliably or consistently available from the patient themselves—like medications, exercise limitations or the results of recent laboratory tests.

Referral information for dietitians:

- reason for referral and expected clinical outcomes
- type and duration of diabetes
- current diabetes management regimen
  - medications (i.e., type, dose, and timing)
  - meal plan, if any
  - exercise guidelines/limitations
  - self-monitoring of glucose records

- medical history
  - height
  - weight
  - age
  - blood pressure
  - other diagnoses and medications prescribed
  - diabetes complications and treatments
- laboratory values
  - glycated hemoglobin A1C
  - glucose values
  - lipid profile
  - microalbumin
- client care goals
- other pertinent information/impressions

The office or clinic where the dietitian practices may have a referral form that prompts the above information. The Nutrition Practice Guidelines include a sample form for referral to MNT (231). For diabetes self-management training, the American Association of Diabetes Educators' *Guide to Reimbursement* provides a ready-to-use referral form (232).

EDUCATIONAL RESOURCES

How do I find nutrition resources to teach and give people with diabetes?

There are a variety of nutrition resources that have been developed for people with diabetes through professional organizations such as the American Diabetes Association (www.diabetes.org), American Dietetic Association (www.eatright.org), the American Association of Diabetes Educators (www.aadenet.org), the Centers for Disease Control and National Institutes of Health National Diabetes Education Program (www.ndep.nih.gov), the National Diabetes Information Clearinghouse (http:// diabetes.niddk.nih.gov/index.htm), and the American Heart Association (www.americanheart.org). Also, there are several health clinics/centers across the country that publish nutrition and diabetes resources (e.g., International Diabetes Center at www.internationaldiabetes center.com, Joslin Clinic at http://www.joslin.harvard. edu/main.shtml). Some resources are free. In addition, many pharmaceutical companies and diabetes-related industries have developed nutrition and diabetes patient education resources that they make available to health care providers, usually at no charge or a minimal cost.

Some specific examples of frequently used resources to teach healthy eating and/or a system of meal planning for people with diabetes are the following, copublished by the American Diabetes Association and the American Dietetic Association.

- *The First Step in Diabetes Meal Planning*
- *Healthy Food Choices*
- *Eating Healthy Foods: Easy Reading Guide*
- *Basic Carbohydrate Counting*
- *Advanced Carbohydrate Counting*

Another resource is *Diabetes: What to Eat*; a publication of the Diabetes Care and Education Practice Group of the American Dietetic Association (available free from Mead Johnson and Company).

I counsel people from a variety of ethnic groups and different cultures. How can I familiarize myself with their food habits, and what resources can I use to teach them about the foods they eat?

Understanding a person's cultural preferences and practices as well as their health and cultural beliefs is important in optimizing the effectiveness of therapy. First, identify the primary cultures of the people you work with. Then seek out resources and/or people that can help you learn about those cultures and their food practices. Consider asking one of your patients to educate you. This can help you demonstrate their value to you. Perhaps you can attend a holiday celebration or a religious service that provides you with insight about their culture. Also try to learn from colleagues who are members of or familiar with particular cultures and their practices.

Ask patients and/or colleagues to share recipes with you. In addition to getting a sense of their nutritional content, you will be able to make suggestions for altering recipes to make them more healthful. It is beneficial to go to the markets where your patients shop or to restaurants that serve their cuisine to have a visual of, learn about, buy, and/or analyze the foods they purchase. Additional information about cultures, food preparation, and recipes is available by doing searches on the Internet and/or using resources available at the local library.

Resources

Holzmeister LA: Nutrition therapy for ethnic populations. In *American Diabetes Association Guide to Medical Nutrition Therapy*. Franz MJ, Bantle JP, Eds. Alexandria, VA, American Diabetes Association, 1999, p. 274–292

Sucher K, Kittler PG: Cultural considerations in diabetes nutrition therapy. In *Handbook of Diabetes Medical Nutrition Therapy*. Powers M, Ed. Gaithersburg, MD, Aspen Publishers, Inc., 1996, p. 284–299

Cultural and Ethnic Food and Nutrition Education Materials, Food and Nutrition Information Center National Agricultural Library, USDA, http://www.nal.usda.gov/fnic/pubs/bibs/gen/ethnic.html

Are there web sites that provide reliable information about nutrition and diabetes?

People with diabetes use the Internet to learn about their disease. It is an incredible tool but can spread false information like wildfire. Caution your patients that

- sites are not regulated for accuracy. Look for reputable sites supported by government, educational institutions, or national organizations such as those listed below.
- sites written by a certified diabetes educator, someone who specializes in both diabetes and nutrition, are more likely to provide reliable content.
- they should not make changes in therapy without consulting their health care team.
- they should be wary of chat room advice and e-mail rumors. Check out rumors (like the aspartame scare) about food, health, and medicine at http://urbanlegends.about.com.

Internet

American Diabetes Association (www.diabetes.org): Includes access to nutrition information, recipes, and publications.

American Dietetic Association (www.eatright.org): Click "Find a Dietitian" to do just that and go to the "Good Nutrition Reading List" for books with reliable information.

American Heart Association (www.americanheart.org): Provides information and resources for the lay public and health professionals.

Tufts University Navigator (www.navigator.tufts.edu): Run by Tufts University, which is well respected for its nutrition know-how. The site rates nutrition-related web sites and helps you find the reliable nutrition sites.

Diabetes 123 (www.diabetes123.com): Offers substantial depth on diabetes topics. Click on "nutrition" to access several useful topics including carb counting, recipes, links to restaurant information, and reviews of diabetes software. Also includes a chat room. Click on Alternative Treatments for a reliable review of dietary supplements.

Calorie King (www.calorieking.com): User-friendly, food-composition database (primarily macronutrients) for 19,000 items

Ashley's Diabetes Information Center (http://206.246.
185.85/diabetes/restaurant.html): Extensive links to
restaurant food composition

The Food and Nutrition Information Center at the US
Department of Agriculture (www.nal.usda.gov/fnic):
Reliable information about food, health, and medicine.
A comprehensive online database is available to search
without charge.

Nutrition.gov (www.nutrition.gov): A clearinghouse for
nutrition information available from the Federal
Government web sites

National Institutes of Health (www.cc.nih.gov/ccc/
supplements/): Facts about dietary supplements

Cyberdiet (www.cyberdiet.com): A member-based,
weight-loss web site run by dietitians. Calculate calories
from food and exercise. Has several record-keeping
tools, menus, shopping lists, and dining out tips.
Posted as $39.95 for 2-month trial or $99.95 for a
year's subscription.

CaloriesCount (www.caloriescount.com): A member-
based, weight-loss web site with reliable information
and good advice. Is similar to Cyberdiet but the
graphics are not as flashy and price is lower ($5/month
and $45 for a year).

Health Success (www.healthsuccess.com): A free site where
diabetes and weight loss hints are exchanged. Hosted by a
well-respected CDE dietitian and author. Includes recipes
and consumer-friendly tips from other readers.

How can I help people with diabetes get the support they need?

Diabetes is difficult enough without trying to manage it
alone. "Support" means what people need to refuel and
keep going. It is what recharges, rather than drains, their
batteries (233).

Although everyone can use support at times, what constitutes support is extremely individual. One person wants someone to listen to them (emotional support) and another needs help with food preparation (practical support). One plays bridge or goes bowling with friends (together), whereas another writes in a journal or reads (alone). One wants a specific meal plan, and another welcomes information and ideas but *not* specific directives. Support doesn't necessarily mean togetherness.

Ask your patients where they get support and what they need or think would help them. Ask what will keep them going, before the novelty of a new regimen wears off. Encourage patients to ask for what they need. Some may need help feeling comfortable or knowing how to ask (assertively) for help. People may find support from:

friends	support groups
family	massage
coworkers	journaling
professional groups	exercise
volunteer groups	ADA
Internet	music
television	spiritual practice
hobbies	workshops
work	helping others
reading	travel
movies	ocean waves
health care team	reflection
counseling	cleaning a closet
playing sports	learning new things
redecorating	theater

Many community diabetes groups or hospital programs offer on-going support or maintenance groups. Participating in Weight Watchers, Overeater's Anonymous, and other nondiabetes meetings can be helpful in maintaining focus, assuming patients may participate using their own diabetes meal plan. The Weight Watcher point system limits calories but does not address quality of intake or carbohydrate distribution. Theoretically, in Overeater's Anonymous (a twelve-step group), members define their own "abstinence," which can easily fit with the lifestyle change goals established with MNT. However, some groups use a preprinted "gray sheet" that is quite specific and restrictive. People who have psychological issues with food, who are depressed, or who have other emotional or mental challenges may need help finding professional resources to address these barriers to lifestyle change. Those who can identify and use their sources of support expand their capacity for making positive behavior changes.

Resources

Rubin RR, Biermann J, Toohey B: *Psyching Out Diabetes.* Los Angeles, Lowell House, 1992

Polonsky WH: *Diabetes Burnout* (on book or audiocassette). Alexandria, VA, American Diabetes Association, 1999

Reimbursement

Because of the Medicare reimbursement guidelines for diabetes education, we are only teaching group classes. How can I effectively individualize a nutrition plan for each person with diabetes in a group setting?

The Medicare reimbursement guidelines include 10 h of education over the course of a year, of which 1 h can be used for a one-to-one appointment for assessment or teaching. The dietitian in the program can use this time to 1) complete a lifestyle assessment, 2) establish initial eating behavioral goals, and 3) develop a "beginning plan of eating."

Those diabetes education programs with dietitians who have completed the application to bill for MNT and received a personal identification number can receive reimbursement for an additional 3 h of MNT above and beyond the 10 h for diabetes self-management training (DSMT) if this service is provided on different days. These visits can be used to provide a more individualized and in-depth plan of eating and/or to revise eating and physical activity behavioral goals as needed.

The remaining 9 h of DSMT must be used for group classes unless the person is unable to attend group classes and meets the Medicare guidelines for one-to-one DSMT. Generally, at least one or two of these hours are used to teach nutrition education. Topics that may be included are nutrition recommendations, planning healthy meals, grocery shopping, reading food labels, and basic carbohydrate counting.

Is MNT and/or diabetes self-management training (DSMT) reimbursed/covered by private payors, managed care, Medicare, and/or Medicaid?

The answers are yes, no, and maybe! To determine whether MNT and/or DSMT are covered benefits, begin by identifying what laws apply to various health plans. Then help patients understand that there are variations in the amount of deductibles, copays, and approved visits as well as variations in who can provide the service and where. Some people are told they have benefits but later find out that MNT/DSMT has to be conducted in a hospital setting and can only be covered after they have met their annual deductible. Some generalities about private payors and managed care are as listed below.

- Some private health plans and managed care organizations are mandated by state laws to cover some MNT and DSMT. Review advocacy information by state on the American Diabetes Association's advocacy web site (www.diabetes.org/advocacy).
- Some health plans do not have to follow state laws because they are so-called ERISA plans. The ERISA (Employee Retirement Insurance Security Act) law, passed in the 1970s, exempts large employee health plans from state health mandates. Some of these plans will cover some DSMT and MNT by choice. What is covered varies from one health plan to the next.
- About 9 million Americans are covered under the Federal Employee Health Benefits plan. These plans are considered ERISA plans and therefore don't have to follow state mandates. Federal Employee Health Benefits represents hundreds of health plans administered by hundreds of health insurance companies. Although coverage of diabetes education and supplies seems to have generally improved, wide variations remain (232).

Note that some of the state laws passed during the last two decades are in jeopardy of being reversed. To learn more, contact the American Diabetes Association or the American Association of Diabetes Educators advocacy staff.

When assisting people who have health coverage through a private payor or managed care plan, encourage them to contact their health plan to determine their benefits for MNT and DSMT. The good news is that more health plans are covering these services. Encourage people to learn how to advocate for themselves to get these very important services covered (see pages 144–145).

Medicaid programs are funded jointly by the states and the Federal government. The Federal government defines benefit categories, such as durable medical equipment (e.g., diabetes supplies). Then, within this broad outline,

each state establishes its own standards and services.
Therefore, both the MNT and DSMT services covered and
the diabetes supplies covered vary from state to state.
Medicaid in each state is usually administered by the state
department of health, welfare, or social services. To determine diabetes benefits, it's best to check with the appropriate department in your state (232).

Medicare is a Federally-funded program that covers
health care expenses for people age ≥65 years, people who
are permanently disabled, and people with end-stage renal
disease. All Medicare beneficiaries receive Part A, which is
in-hospital services, including medications. Medicare
beneficiaries can choose to get Part B and pay a monthly
premium. Part B covers professional services. DSMT,
MNT, and diabetes supplies are covered under Part B,
and lengthy regulations apply to all three benefits. Several
diabetes-related organizations have partnered to provide
web-based resources on these regulations (226–229). To
learn more about Medicare, visit www.medicare. gov. It is
also common for people on Medicare to have a supplemental health plan. This is particularly useful to cover
pharmaceutical expenses, because at press these are not
covered outside of the hospital under Medicare. A person's MNT and/or DSMT may be covered under his or
her supplemental plan in full or in part (226–232).

Does the nutrition service(s) provided within a diabetes self-management training (DSMT) program and reimbursed by Medicare differ from the nutrition service(s) provided by a dietitian as MNT and reimbursed by Medicare?

DSMT and MNT are viewed by Medicare as distinct but
complementary benefits (234). The only stipulation is that
they may not be *provided* on the same date of service. They
can, however, be *billed* on the same date of service. In

coordinating the DSMT and MNT services, Medicare differentiates the nutrition services provided in DSMT and MNT as follows:

The DSMT benefit consists of ten different functional areas (curriculum content areas) of which nutrition counseling is only one. The intent of DSMT is to provide overall guidance related to all aspects of the disease to increase the beneficiary's knowledge about the disease and how they can exercise control over their own health. Medicare describes MNT as a more intensive nutritional counseling and therapy regimen that relies heavily on follow-up and feedback to the beneficiary to change their behavior over a period of time (234,226). The rationale used in the Medicare regulations for covering both DSMT and MNT is that the two benefits provide different behavioral modification techniques, which may prove to be complementary. This coverage policy was adopted to allow the Medicare beneficiary to receive the effect of reinforcement over a period of time.

Do health plans reimburse for medical care, MNT, and diabetes self-management training (DSMT) for a person who has pre-diabetes and/or metabolic syndrome?

Pre-diabetes has been defined as fasting blood glucose ≥110–125 mg/dl (impaired fasting glucose) or blood glucose ≥140–199 mg/dl on a 2-h oral glucose tolerance test (impaired glucose tolerance). It has been suggested that the oral glucose tolerance test appears to identify more people who have impaired glucose homeostasis and thus, more people who will progress to diabetes (218). Metabolic syndrome has been defined as having at least three of the following:

■ waist circumference >102 cm (40") in men, >88 cm (35") in women
■ serum triglycerides >150 mg/dl

- high-density lipoprotein <40 mg/dl in men, <50 mg/dl in women
- blood pressure >130/85
- serum glucose level >110 mg/dl (235)

Clearly, many individuals who have pre-diabetes also have metabolic syndrome and thus meet the above noted criteria.

The only ICD-9 code that exists for pre-diabetes at present is 790.2, for impaired glucose tolerance (236). Another ICD-9 code 277.7 was recently added, for the dysmetabolic syndrome. To utilize code 277.7 for reimbursement, the person should have at least 3 of the 5 variables listed above for metabolic syndrome. As this code is relatively new, diabetes care providers might want to check with private payers about whether they recognize this code alone, or whether using the individual three appropriate codes is preferred.

These two ICD-9 codes may be helpful in providing medical care, MNT, and DSMT to people with pre-diabetes and/or metabolic syndrome. To date, coverage from private payors using these codes is variable. Using good business practices can improve coverage for MNT and DSMT. These include obtaining appropriate referral information, setting appropriate fees, maintaining appropriate records and documentation, correctly billing for services provided, and measuring effectiveness outcomes (237). In many cases, people with pre-diabetes and/or metabolic syndrome have related billable diagnoses, such as hypertension and dyslipidemia. These can assist in reimbursement for medical care, MNT, and DSMT. Although some private payers may not recognize the above noted codes as a billable service, coverage is at least occasionally provided. Diabetes care providers should collect data on coverage in their practices.

It's important to keep in mind that new ground is being paved regarding reimbursement for pre-diabetes and metabolic syndrome. Do keep in mind, however, that there is substantial evidence that the implementation of lifestyle interventions for individuals with pre-diabetes can prevent and/or delay the onset of diabetes (218,139,140). It may be useful to use this data when seeking reimbursement for your services.

At present, the Medicare regulations for MNT and DSMT do not include coverage of these services for people with pre-diabetes or metabolic syndrome. People must have the diagnosis of diabetes for MNT and must qualify with even more stringent criteria for DSMT (226–229). Individuals who believe criteria for MNT and DSMT should include pre-diabetes are urged to work with their Federal legislators and diabetes-related organizations to initiate a legislative change in the current Medicare regulations to include coverage of MNT and DSMT for people with pre-diabetes.

Does insurance reimburse for MNT to treat obesity?

Coverage and reimbursement strategies for obesity are changing in large part because of cost pressures, consumer demand, and the greater attention being paid to evidence-based medicine (238). Generally, medical care for obesity treatment per se is not covered by private payers, and neither is MNT for weight reduction. However, health risk assessments are increasingly being used to profile patients who would benefit from disease management strategies that may include nutrition interventions (238).

When other health conditions are present, such as diabetes, hypertension, or dyslipidemia, which is quite common, the possibility of reimbursement for medical care and MNT is improved (see pages 158–160). Some health plans make coverage decisions based on individual patient situations, whereas others have a set policy regardless of who the patient is and what their medical conditions are.

Portions of medical care that are most likely to be eligible for coverage for obese people with other medical problems are physician visits and lab work. Private payers do not reimburse for lifestyle change education, meal replacement formulas, or nutritional supplements used for obesity treatment. Prescriptions for obesity medications are also rarely covered.

With regard to the coverage for bariatric surgery for the treatment of obesity, some health plans provide coverage when certain conditions and criteria are met. The patient would have to meet the medical criteria outlined in literature as being necessary to qualify for bariatric surgery. In addition, health plans typically require documentation that the patient has participated in, but without success, a physician-directed weight loss program. The cost of gastric surgery for obesity varies, but ranges between $15,000 and $50,000 initially.

References

1. American Diabetes Association: Evidence-based nutrition principles and recommendations for the treatment and prevention of diabetes and related complications (Position Statement). *Diabetes Care* 26 (Suppl. 1):S51–S61, 2003

2. Franz MJ, Bantle JP, Beebe CA, Brunzell JD, Chiasson JL, Garg A, Holzmeister LA, Hoogwerf B, Mayer-Davis E, Mooradian AD, Purnell JQ, Wheeler M: Evidence-based nutrition principles and recommendations for the treatment and prevention of diabetes and related complications (Technical Review). *Diabetes Care* 25(1):148–198, 2002

3. UK Prospective Diabetes Study 7: Response of fasting plasma glucose to diet therapy in newly presenting type II diabetic patients. *Metabolism* 39:905–912, 1990

4. Franz MJ, Monk A, Barry B, McClain K, Weaver T, Cooper N, Upham P, Bergenstal R, Mazze RS: Effectiveness of medical nutrition therapy provided by dietitians in the management of non-insulin-dependent diabetes mellitus: a randomized, controlled clinical trial. *J Am Diet Assoc* 95:1009–1017, 1995

5. Kulkarni K, Castle G, Gregory R, Holmes A, Leontos C, Powers M, Snetselaar L, Splett P, Wylie-Rosett J: Nutrition practice guidelines for type 1 diabetes mellitus positively affect dietitian practices and patient outcomes. *J Am Diet Assoc* 98:62–70, 1998

6. Appel LJ, Moore TJ, Obarzanek E, Vollmer VW, Svetkey LP, Sacks FM, Bray GA, Vogt TM, Cutler JA, Windhauser MM, Lin PH, Karanja N: A clinical trial of the effects of dietary patterns on blood pressure. *N Engl J Med* 336:1117–1124, 1997

7. Kant AK, Schatzkin A, Graubard BI, Schairer C: A prospective study of diet quality and mortality in women. *JAMA* 283:2109–2115, 2000

8. Huijbregts P, Feskens E, Rasanen L, Fidanza F, Nissinen A, Menotti A, Kromhout D: Dietary patterns and 20 year mortality in elderly men in Finland, Italy, and The

Netherlands: longitudinal cohort study. *BMJ* 315:13–17, 1997

9. Krauss RM, Eckel RH, Howard B, Appel LJ, Daniels SR, Deckelbaum RJ, Erdman JW, Kris-Etherton P, Goldberg IJ, Kotchen TA, Lichtenstein AH, Mitch WE, Mullis R, Robinson K, Wylie-Rosett J, St Jeor S, Suttie J, Tribble DL, Bazzarre TL: AHA dietary guidelines. Revision 2000: a statement for healthcare professionals from the nutrition committee of the American Heart Association. *Circulation* 102:2284–2299, 2000

10. U.S. Department of Agriculture, U.S. Department of Health and Human Services: *Nutrition and Your Health: Dietary Guidelines for Americans.* 5th ed. Home and Garden Bulletin No. 232, 2000

11. Expert Panel on Detection, Evaluation, and Treatment of High Blood Cholesterol in Adults: Executive summary of the third report of the National Cholesterol Education Program (NCEP) expert panel on detection, evaluation, and treatment of high blood cholesterol in adults (Adult Treatment Panel III). *JAMA* 285:2486–2497, 2001

12. National Heart, Lung, and Blood Institute Joint National Committee on Prevention, Detection, Evaluation, and Treatment of High Blood Pressure: The 7th report of the Joint National Committee on Prevention, Detection, Evaluation, and Treatment of High Blood Pressure: the JNC 7 report. *JAMA* 289:2560–2572, 2003

13. Green Pastors J, Warshaw H, Daly A, Franz M, Kulkarni K: The evidence for the effectiveness of medical nutrition therapy in diabetes management. *Diabetes Care* 25:608–613, 2002

14. Green Pastors J, Franz M, Warshaw H, Daly A, Arnold M: How effective is diabetes medical nutrition therapy? *J Am Diet Assoc* 103:827–831, 2003

15. DAFNE Study Group: Training in flexible, intensive insulin management to enable dietary freedom in people with type 1 diabetes: dose adjustment for normal eating (DAFNE) randomized controlled trial. *BMJ* 325:746–752, 2002

16. Kris-Etherton PM, Yu S: Individual fatty acids effects on plasma lipids and lipoproteins: human studies. *Am J Clin Nutr* 6 (Suppl. 5):1628S–1644S, 1997

17. Yu-Poth S, Zhao G, Etherton T, Naglak M, Jonnalagadda S, Kris-Etherton PM: Effects of the National Cholesterol Education Program's Step I and Step II dietary intervention programs on cardiovascular disease risk factors: a meta-analysis. *Am J Clin Nutr* 69:632–646, 1999

18. American Diabetes Association: Management of dyslipidemia in adults with diabetes (Position Statement). *Diabetes Care* 26 (Suppl. 1): S83–S86, 2003

19. Cutler JA, Follmann D, Allender PS: Randomized trials of sodium restriction: an overview. *Am J Clin Nutr* 65 (Suppl. 1):643S–651S, 1997

20. Sacks FM, Svetkey LP, Vollmer WM, Appel LJ, Bray GA, Harsha D, Obarzanek E, Conlin PR, Miller ER, Simons-Morton DG, Karanja N, Lin P-H for the DASH-Sodium Collaborative Research Group: Effects on blood pressure of reduced dietary sodium and the dietary approaches to stop hypertension (DASH) diet. *New Engl J Med* 344(1):3–10, 2001

21. Stamler R, Stamler J, Gosch FC, Civinelli J, Fishman J, McKeever P, McDonald A, Dyer AR: Primary prevention of hypertension by nutritional-hygienic means: final report of a randomized, controlled trial. *JAMA* 262:1801–1807, 1989

22. Institute of Medicine's Food and Nutrition Board: *Dietary Reference Intakes for Energy, Carbohydrate, Fiber, Fat, Fatty Acids, Cholesterol, Protein, and Amino Acids.* Washington, DC, National Academies Press, 2002

23. Report of a Joint FAO/WHO Expert Consultation: *Carbohydrates in Human Nutrition.* Rome, Italy, Food and Agriculture Organization of the United Nations and World Health Organization, 1998

24. Wolever TMS, Nguyen PM, Chiasson JL, Hunt JA, Josse RG, Palmason C, Rodger NW, Ross SA, Ryan EA, Tan MH: Determinants or diet glycemic index calculated retrospectively from diet records of 342 individuals with non-insulin-dependent diabetes mellitus. *Am J Clin Nutr* 59:1265–1269, 1994

25. Crapo PA, Reaven G, Olefsky J: Postprandial plasma-glucose and insulin responses to different complex carbohydrates. *Diabetes* 26:1178–1183, 1977

26. Bantle JP, Laine DC, Castle GW, Thomas W, Hoogwerf BJ, Goetz FC: Postprandial glucose and insulin responses to meals containing different carbohydrates in normal and diabetic subjects. *N Engl J Med* 309:7–12, 1983

27. Franz MJ: Carbohydrate and diabetes: is the source or the amount of more importance? *Diabetes Current Concepts* 1:177–186, 2001

28. Garg A, Bantle JP, Henry RR, Coulston AN, Griver KA, Raatz SK, Brinkley L, Chen YD, Grunday SM, Huet BA: Effects of varying carbohydrate content of diet in patients with non-insulin-dependent diabetes mellitus. *JAMA* 271:1421–1428, 1994

29. Heilbronn L, Noakes M, Clifton P: Effect of energy restriction, weight loss, and diet composition on plasma lipids and glucose in patients with type 2 diabetes. *Diabetes Care* 22:889–895, 1999

30. Eely EA, Stratton IM, Hadden DR, on behalf of the UKPDS: Estimated dietary intake in type 2 diabetic patients randomly allocated to diet, sulfonylurea, or insulin therapy (UKPDS). *Diabetic Med* 13:656–662, 1996

31. Yang EJ, Chung HK, Kim WY, Kerver JM, Song WG: Carbohydrate intake is associated with diet quality and risk factors for cardiovascular disease in U.S. adults: NHANES III. *J Am Coll Nutr* 22:71–79, 2002

32. Turley ML, Skeaff CM, Mann JI, Cox B: The effect of a low-fat, high-carbohydrate diet on serum high density lipoprotein cholesterol and triglyceride. *Eur J Clin Nutr* 52:728–732, 1998

33. Toubro S, Astrup A: Randomized comparison of diet for maintaining obese subjects' weight after major weight loss: ad lib, low fat, high carbohydrate diet vs. fixed energy intake. *BMJ* 314:29–34, 1997

34. Jenkins DJ, Wolever TM, Taylor RH, Barker H, Fielden H, Baldwin JM, Bowling AC, Newman HC, Jenkins AL, Goff DV: Glycemic index of foods: a physiological basis for carbohydrate exchange. *Am J Clin Nutr* 34:362–366, 1981

35. Wolever TM, Jenkins DJ, Jenkins AL, Josse RG: The glycemic index: methodology and clinical implications. *Am J Clin Nutr* 54:846–854, 1991

36. Ludwig DS: Dietary glycemic index and obesity. *J Nutr* 130 (Suppl.):280S–283S, 1990

37. Pi-Sunyer FX: Glycemic index and disease. *Am J Clin Nutr* 76 (Suppl.):290S–298S, 2002

38. Brand-Miller J, Hayne S, Petocz P, Colagiuri S: Low glycemic index diets in the management of diabetes: a meta-analysis of randomized controlled trials. *Diabetes Care* 26:2261–2267, 2003

39. Franz MJ: The glycemic index: not the most effective nutrition therapy intervention. *Diabetes Care* 26:2466–2468, 2003

40. Coulston AM, Hollenbeck CB, Liu GC, Williams RA, Starich GH, Mazzaferri EL, Reaven GM: Effect of source of dietary carbohydrate on plasma glucose, insulin, and gastric inhibitory polypeptide responses to test meals in subjects with noninsulin-dependent diabetes mellitus. *Am J Clin Nutr* 40:975–970, 1984

41. Wolever TMS, Jenkins DJA: The use of the glycemic index in predicting the blood glucose response to mixed meals. *Am J Clin Nutr* 44:167–172, 1986

42. Foster-Powell K, Holt SHA, Brand-Miller JC: International tables of glycemic load values: 2002. *Am J Clin Nutr* 76:5–56, 2002

43. Warshaw HS, Powers MA: A search for answers about foods with polyols (sugar alcohols). *The Diabetes Educator* 25(3):307–319, 1999

44. Powers MA: Sugar alternatives and fat replacers. In *American Diabetes Association Guide to Medical Nutrition Therapy.* Franz MJ, Bantle JP, Eds. Alexandria, VA, American Diabetes Association, 1999, pp. 148–164

45. National Institutes of Environmental Health Sciences: *9th National Toxicology Report on Carcinogens.* Washington, DC, DHHS, NIH, May 2000

46. Lafrance L, Rabasa-Lhoret R, Poisson D, Ducros F, Chiasson J-L: Effects of different glycemic index foods and dietary fibre intake on glyceaemic control in type 1 dia-

betic patients on intensive insulin therapy. *Diabetic Medicine* 15:972–978, 1998

47. Giacco R, Parillo M, Rivellese AA, Lasorella G, Giacco A, D'Episcopo L, Riccardi G: Long-term dietary treatment with increased amounts of fiber-rich low-glycemic index natural foods improved blood glucose control and reduces the number of hypoglycemic events in type 1 diabetic patients. *Diabetes Care* 23:1461–1466, 2000

48. Hollenbeck CB, Coulston AM, Reaven GM: To what extent does increased dietary fiber improve glucose and lipid metabolism in patients with non-insulin-dependent diabetes mellitus (NIDDM)? *Am J Clin Nutr* 43:16–24, 1986

49. Chandalia M, Garg A, Lutjohann D, Bergmann KV, Grundy SM, Brinkley LJ: Beneficial effects of high dietary fiber intake in patients with type 2 diabetes mellitus. *N Engl J Med* 342:1392–1398, 2000

50. Brown L, Rosner B, Willett WW, Sacks FM: Cholesterol-lowering effects of dietary fiber: a meta-analysis. *Am J Clin Nutr* 69:30–43, 1999

51. American Cancer Society: Can colon and rectum cancer be prevented? American Cancer Society, http://www.cancer.org/docroot/CRI/content/CRI_2_4_2X_Can_colon_and_rectum_cancer_be_prevented.asp?sitearea. (accessed February 25, 2003)

52. Conn JW, Newburgh LH: The glycemic response to isoglucogenic quantities of protein and carbohydrate. *J Clin Invest* 15:667–671, 1936

53. Nuttall FQ, Mooradian AD, Gannon MC, Billington C, Krezowski P: Effect of protein ingestion on the glucose and insulin response to a standardized oral glucose load. *Diabetes Care* 7:465–470, 1984

54. Gannon MC, Nuttall JA, Damberg G, Gupta V, Nuttall FQ: Effect of protein ingestion on the glucose appearance rate in people with type 2 diabetes. *J Clin Endocrinol Metab* 86:1040–1047, 2001

55. Fajan SS, Floyd JC, Pek S, Knopf RF, Jacobson M, Conn JW: Effect of protein meals on plasma insulin in mildly diabetic individuals. *Diabetes* 18:523–528, 1969

56. Franz MJ: Protein and diabetes: much advice, little research. *Current Diabetes Reports* 2:457–464, 2002

57. Gougeon R, Pencharz PB, Sigal RJ: Effect of glycemic control on the kinetics of whole-body protein metabolism in obese subjects with non-insulin dependent diabetes mellitus during iso and hypoenergetic feeding. *Am J Clin Nutr* 65:861–870, 1997

58. Pacy PJ, Nair KS, Ford C, Halliday D: Failure of insulin infusion to stimulate fractional muscle protein synthesis in type 1 diabetic patients: anabolic effects of insulin and decreased proteolysis. *Diabetes* 38:618–624, 1989

59. Gougeon R, Pencharz PB, Marliss EB: Effects of NIDDM on the kinetics of whole-body protein metabolism. *Diabetes* 43:318–328, 1994

60. Hofer LF: Are dietary protein requirements altered in diabetes mellitus? *Can J Physiol Pharmacol* 71:633–638, 1993

61. Toeller M, Buyken A, Heitkamp G, Bramswig S, Mann J, Milne R, Gries FA, Keen H, and the EURODIAB IDDM Complications Study Group: Protein intake and urinary albumin excretion rates in the EURODIAB IDDM Complications Study. *Diabetologia* 40:1219–1226, 1997

62. Wrone EM, Carnethon MR, Palaniappan L, Fortmann SP: Association of dietary protein intake and microalbuminuria in health adults. *Am J Kidney Dis* 41:580–587, 2003

63. Wheeler ML: Nephropathy and medical nutrition therapy. In *American Diabetes Association Guide to Medical Nutrition Therapy for Diabetes.* Franz MJ, Bantle JP, Eds. Alexandria, VA, American Diabetes Association, 1999, pp. 312–323

64. Zeller K, Whittaker E, Sullivan L, Raskin P, Jacobson HR: Effect of restricting dietary protein on the progression of renal disease in patients with insulin-dependent diabetes. *N Engl J Med* 324:78–84, 1991

65. Walker JD, Bending JJ, Dodds RA, Mattock MB, Murrells TJ, Keen H, Viberti GC: Restriction of dietary protein and progression of renal failure in diabetic nephropathy. *Lancet* ii:1411–1415, 1989

66. Meloni C, Morosetti M, Suraci C, Pennafina MG, Tozzo C, Taccone-Gallucci M, Casciani CU: Severe dietary pro-

tein restriction in overt diabetic nephropathy: benefits or risks? *J Renal Nutr* 12:96–101, 2002

67. Wheeler ML, Fineberg SE, Fineberg NS, Gibson RG, Hackward LL: Animal versus plant protein meals in individuals with type 2 diabetes and microalbuminuria. *Diabetes Care* 15:1277–1282, 2002

68. Ruderman N, Chisholm D, Pi-Sunyer X, Schneider S: The metabolically obese, normal-weight individual revisited. *Diabetes* 47:699–713, 1998

69. Bessessen DH: The role of carbohydrates in insulin resistance. *J Nutr* 131:2782S–2786S, 2001

70. Daly ME, Vale C, Walker M, Alberti KGMM, Mathers JC: Dietary carbohydrates and insulin sensitivity: a review of the evidence and clinical implications. *Am J Clin Nutr* 66:1072–1095, 1997

71. Lovejoy JC: The influence of dietary fat on insulin resistance. *Current Diabetes Reports* 2:435–440, 2002

72. Louheranta AM, Schwab US, Sarkkinen ES: Insulin sensitivity after a reduced-fat diet and a monene-enriched diet in subjects with elevated serum cholesterol and triglyceride concentrations. *Nutr Metab Cardiovasc Dis* 10:177–187, 2000

73. Goodyear LJ, Kahn BB: Exercise, glucose transport, and insulin sensitivity. *Ann Rev Med* 49: 235–261, 1998

74. Krauss RM, Eckel RH, Howard B, Appel LJ, Daniels SR, Deckelbaum RJ, Erdman JW, Kris-Etherton P, Goldberg IJ, Kotchen TA, Lichtenstein AH, Mitch WE, Mullis R, Robinson K, Wylie-Rosett J, St Jeor S, Suttie J, Tribble DL, Bazzarre TL: AHA dietary guidelines. Revision 2000: a statement for healthcare professionals from the nutrition committee of the American Heart Association. *Circulation* 102:2284–2299, 2000

75. Expert Panel on Detection, Evaluation, and Treatment of High Blood Cholesterol in Adults: Executive summary of the third report of the National Cholesterol Education Program (NCEP) expert panel on detection, evaluation, and treatment of high blood cholesterol in adults (Adult Treatment Panel III). *JAMA* 285:2486–2497, 2001

76. Franz MJ: So many nutrition recommendations—contradictory or compatible? *Diabetes Spectrum* 16:56–63, 2003

77. Lovejoy JC, DiGirolamo M: Habitual dietary intake and insulin sensitivity in lean and obese adults. *Am J Clin Nutr* 55:1174–1749, 1992

78. Parillo M, Rivellese AA, Ciardullo AV, Capaldo B, Giacco A, Genovese S, Ricardi G: A high-monounsaturated fat/low carbohydrate diet improves peripheral insulin sensitivity in non-insulin-dependent diabetic patients. *Metabolism* 41:1373–1378, 1992

79. Lichtenstein AH, Ausman LM, Carrasco W, Jenner JL, Ordovas JM, Schaefer EJ: Short-term consumption of a low fat diet beneficially affects plasma lipid concentrations only when accompanied by weight loss. *Arterioscler Thromb* 14:1751–1760, 1994

80. Carmichael HE, Swinburn BA, Wilson MR: Lower fat intake as a predictor of initial and sustained weight loss in obese subjects consuming an otherwise ad libitum diet. *J Am Diet Assoc* 98:35–39, 1998

81. Astrup A, Ryan L, Grunwald GK, Storgaard M, Saris W, Melanson E, Hill JO: The role of dietary fat in body fatness: evidence from a preliminary meta-analysis of ad libitum low-fat dietary intervention study. *Br J Nutr* 83 (Suppl. 1):S25–S32, 2000

82. Franz, MJ: *Exchanges for All Occasions. Your Guide to Choosing Healthy Foods Anytime Anywhere.* Minneapolis, MN, IDC Publishing, 1997

83. Sigman-Grant M: Can you have your low-fat cake and eat it too? The role of fat-modified products. *J Am Diet Assoc* 97(7):S76–S81, 1997

84. Carter NB: Plant stanol esters: review of cholesterol lowering efficacy and implications for CHD risk reduction. *Prev Card* 3:121–130, 2000

85. Blair SN, Capuzzi DM, Gottleib SO, Nguyen T, Morgan JM, Cater NB: Incremental reduction of serum total cholesterol and low-density lipoprotein cholesterol with the addition of plant stanol ester-containing spread to statin therapy. *Am J Cardiol* 86:46–52, 2000

86. Hu FB, Eunyoung C, Rexrode KM, Albert CM, and Manson JE: Fish and long-chain omega-3 fatty acid intake and risk of coronary heart disease and total mortality in diabetic women. *Circulation* 107:1852–1857, 2003

87. Dunstan DW, Mori TA, Puddey IB: The independent and combined effects of aerobic exercise and dietary fish intake on serum lipids and glycemic control in NIDDM: a randomized, controlled study. *Diabetes Care* 20:913–921, 1997

88. Friedberg CE, Janssen MJFM, Heine RJ: Fish oil and glycemic control in diabetes: a meta-analysis. *Diabetes Care* 21:494–500, 1998

89. Montori VM, Farmer A, Wollan PC: Fish oil supplementation in type 2 diabetes: a quantitative systematic review. *Diabetes Care* 23:1407–1415, 2000

90. Frezza M, di Padova C, Pozzato G, Terpin M, Baraona E, Lieber CS: High blood alcohol levels in women. The role of decreased gastric alcohol dehydrogenase activity and first-pass metabolism. *N Engl J Med* 322:95–99, 1990

91. Koivisto VA, Tulokas S, Toivonen M, Haapa E, Pelkonen R: Alcohol with meal has no adverse effects on postprandial glucose homeostasis in patients with diabetes. *Diabetes Care* 16(12):1612–1614, 1993

92. Ben G, Gnidi L, Maran A, Gigante A, Duner E, Iori E, Tiengo A, Avogaro A: Effects of chronic alcohol intake on carbohydrate and lipid metabolism in subjects with type II (non-insulin-dependent) diabetes. *Am J Med* 90:70–76, 1991

93. Turner BC, Jenkins E, Kerr D, Sherwin RS, Cavan DA: The effect of evening alcohol consumption on next-morning glucose control in type 1 diabetes. *Diabetes Care* 24:1889–1893, 2001

94. Wei M, Gibbon LW, Mitchell TL, Kampert JB, Blair SN: Alcohol intake and incidence of type 2 diabetes in men. *Diabetes Care* 23:18–22, 2000

95. Ajani UA, Hennekens CH, Spelsberg A, Manson JE: Alcohol consumption and risk of type 2 diabetes mellitus among U.S. male physicians. *Arch Intern Med* 160:1025–1030, 2000

96. Valmadrid CT, Klein R, Moss SE, Klein BK, Cruickshanks KJ: Alcohol intake and the risk of coronary heart disease mortality in persons with older-onset diabetes. *JAMA* 282:239–246, 1999

97. Ajani UA, Gaziano JM, Lotufo PA, Liu S, Hennekens CH, Buring JE, Manson JE: Alcohol consumption and risk of coronary heart disease by diabetes status. *Circulation* 102:500–505, 2000

98. Sacco RL, Elkind M, Boden-Albala B, Lin IF, Kargman DE, Hauser WA, Shea D, Paik MC: The protective effect of moderate alcohol consumption on ischemic stroke. *JAMA* 281:53–60, 1999

99. Facchini F, Chen Y-D, Reaven GM: Light-to-moderate alcohol intake is associated with insulin sensitivity. *Diabetes Care* 17:115–119, 1994

100. Davies MJ, Baer DJ, Judd JT, Brown ED, Campbell WS, Taylor PR: Effects of moderate alcohol intake on fasting insulin and glucose concentrations and insulin sensitivity in postmenopausal women. *JAMA* 287:2559–2562, 2002

101. Nanchahal K, Ashton WD, Wood DA: Alcohol consumption, metabolic cardiovascular risk factors and hypertension in women. *Int J Epidemiol* 29:57–64, 2000

102. Joint National Committee on Prevention, Detection, Evaluation and Treatment of High Blood Pressure: The sixth report of the Joint National Committee on Prevention, Detection, Evaluation, and Treatment of high blood pressure. *Arch Intern Med* 157:2143–2446, 1997

103. Israelsson B: Role of alcohol, glucose intolerance and obesity in hypertriglyceridemia. *Atherosclerosis* 62:123–127, 1986

104. Pownall HJ, Ballantyne CH, Kimball KT, Simpson SL, Yeshurum D, Grotto AM: Effect of moderate alcohol consumption on hypertriglyceridemia. *Arch Intern Med* 159:981, 1999

105. Franz MJ: Alcohol and diabetes. In *American Diabetes Association Guide to Medical Nutrition Therapy for Diabetes.* Franz MJ, Bantle JP, Eds. Alexandria, VA: American Diabetes Association, 1999, pp.192–208

106. McWhorter L, Geil P: Interactions between complementary therapies or nutrition supplements and conventional medications *Diabetes Spectrum* 16:262–266, 2002

107. Institute of Medicine: *Dietary Reference Intakes for Vitamin C, Vitamin E, Selenium, and Carotenoids.* Washington, DC, National Academy Press, 2000

108. Hasanain B, Mooradian AD: Antioxidant vitamins and their influence in diabetes mellitus. *Current Diabetes Reports* 2:448–456, 2002

109. Vivekananthan DP, Penn MS, Sapp SK, Hsu A, Topol EJ: Use of antioxidant vitamins for the prevention of cardiovascular disease: meta-analysis of randomized trials. *Lancet* 361:2017–2033, 2003

110. Omenn GS, Goodman GE, Thornquist MD: Risk factors for lung cancer and for intervention effects in CARET: the Beta Carotene and Retinol Efficacy Trial. *J Natl Cancer Inst* 88:1550–1559, 1996

111. The Alpha-Tocopherol, Beta Carotene Cancer Prevention Study Group: The effect of vitamin E and beta carotene on the incidence of lung cancer and other cancers in male smokers. *N Engl J Med* 330:1029–1035, 1994

112. Lonn E, Yusuf S, Hoogwerf B, Pogue J, Yi Q, Zinman B, Bosch J, Dagenais G, Mann JFE, Cerstein DC, on behalf of the Heart Outcomes Prevention Evaluation (HOPE) Investigators: Effects of vitamin E on cardiovascular and microvascular outcomes in high-risk patients with diabetes. *Diabetes Care* 25:1919–1927, 2002

113. Waters DD, Alderman EL, Hsia J, Howard BV, Cobb FH, Rogers WJ, Ouyang P, Thompson P, Tardif JC, Higginson L, Bittner V, Steffes M, Gordon DJ, Proschan M, Younes N, Verter JL: Effects of hormone replacements and antioxidant vitamin supplements on coronary atherosclerosis in postmenopausal women. A randomized controlled trial. *JAMA* 288:2432–2440, 2002

114. Brown BG, Zhao XQ, Chait A, Albers JJ, Brown BG: Antioxidant supplements block the response of HDL to simvastatin-niacin therapy in patients with coronary artery disease and low HDL. *N Engl J Med* 345:1583–1592, 2001

115. American Diabetes Association: Treatment of hypertension in adults with diabetes (Position Statement). *Diabetes Care* 26 (Suppl. 1):S80–82, 2002

116. Aronne LJ: Treatment of obesity in the primary care setting. In *Handbook of Obesity Treatment.* Wadden T, Stunkard AJ, Eds. New York, Guilford Press, 2002, pp.383–394

117. Ruggiero L: Helping people with diabetes change behavior: from theory to practice. *Diabetes Spectrum* 13:125–132, 2002

118. Brownell KD, Wadden TA: *The LEARN Program for Weight Control: Special Medication Addition.* Dallas, TX, American Health, 1998

119. National Heart, Lung and Blood Institute (NHLBI) Obesity Education Initiative Expert Panel on the Identification, Evaluation, and Treatment of Overweight and Obesity in Adults: *Clinical guidelines on the identification, evaluation, and treatment of overweight and obesity in adults: the evidence report.* Bethesda, MD, National Institutes of Health, 1998, (NIH publ. no. 98-4083)

120. American Diabetes Association: Standards of medical care for patients with diabetes mellitus (Position Statement). *Diabetes Care* 26:S33–50, 2003

121. Siminerio L, McLaughlin S, Polonsky W: *Diabetes Education Goals,* 3rd ed. American Diabetes Association, Alexandria, VA, 2003

122. American Diabetes Association: National standards for diabetes self-management education (Standards and Review Criteria). *Diabetes Care* 26:S149–S156, 2003

123. Green Pastors J: Process of diabetes medical nutrition therapy. In *Diabetes Medical Nutrition Therapy.* Holler H, Green Pastors J, Eds. American Dietetic Association/American Diabetes Association, Chicago/Alexandria, VA, 1997

124. American Diabetes Association: Translation of the diabetes nutrition recommendations for health care institutions (Position Statement). *Diabetes Care* 26:S70–S72, 2003

125. Diabetes Control and Complications Trial Research Group: The effect of intensive treatment of diabetes on the

development and progression of long-term complications in insulin-dependent diabetes mellitus. *N Engl J Med* 329:977–986, 1993

126. UK Prospective Diabetes Study Group: Intensive blood-glucose control with sulphonylureas or insulin compared with conventional treatment and risk of complications in patients with type 2 diabetes (UKPDS33). *Lancet* 352:837–853,1998

127. Diabetes Control and Complications Trial Research Group: Nutrition interventions for intensive therapy in the Diabetes Control and Complications Trial. *J Am Diet Assoc* 93:768–762, 1993

128. American Diabetes Association: Continuous subcutaneous infusion of insulin (Position Statement). *Diabetes Care* 26 (Suppl. 1):S125, 2003

129. Daly A, Gillespie S, Kulkarni K: Carbohydrate counting: vignettes from the trenches. *Diabetes Spectrum* 9:114–117, 1996

130. Gillespie SJ, Kulkarni K, Daly AE: Using carbohydrate counting in diabetes clinical practice. *J Am Diet Assoc* 98:897–905, 1998

131. Warshaw HS, Bolderman KM: *Practical Carbohydrate Counting.* American Diabetes Association, Alexandria, VA, 2001

132. American Diabetes Association, American Dietetic Association: *Basic Carbohydrate Counting.* Alexandria, VA, American Diabetes Association/Chicago, American Dietetic Association, 2003

133. American Diabetes Association, American Dietetic Association: *Advanced Carbohydrate Counting.* Alexandria, VA, American Diabetes Association/Chicago, American Dietetic Association, 2003

134. Daly A, Franz M, Holzmeister LA, Kulkarni K, O'Connell B, Wheeler M: New diabetes nutrition resources. *J Am Diet Assoc,* 103:832–834, 2003

135. Franz M, Reader D, Monk A: *Implementing Group and Individual Medical Nutrition Therapy for Diabetes.* American Diabetes Association, Alexandria, VA, 2002

136. Franz MJ, Green Pastors J, Warshaw H, Daly AE: Does "diet" fail? *Diabetes Educator* 27:563–569, 2001

137. VanWormer JF, Boucher JL: Motivational interviewing and diabetes education: fostering commitment to change in facilitating behavior change. *On The Cutting Edge* 24:14–16, 2003

138. Brackenridge B: Discovery learning: a behavioral approach to meal planning in facilitating behavior change. *On The Cutting Edge* 24:11–13, 2003

139. Diabetes Prevention Research Group: Reduction in the evidence of type 2 diabetes with lifestyle intervention or metformin. *N Engl J Med* 346:393–403, 2002

140. Tuomilehto J, Lindstrom J, Eriksson JG, Valle TT, Hamalainen H, Ilanne-Parikks P, Keinanen-Kiukaanniemi S, Laakso M, Louheranta A, Rastas M, Salminen V, Uusitupa M; Finnish Diabetes Prevention Study Group: Prevention of type 2 diabetes mellitus by changes in lifestyle among subjects with impaired glucose tolerance. *N Engl J Med* 344:1343–1350, 2001

141. Green Pastors J, Franz MJ, Warshaw H, Daly A, Arnold M: How effective is medical nutrition therapy in diabetes care. *J Am Diet Assoc* 103:827–831, 2003

142. Peeples M, Mulcahy K, Tomky D, Weaver T: The conceptual framework of the National Diabetes Education Outcomes System (NDEOS). *Diabetes Educator* 27:547–562, 2001

143. Franz M: Exercise benefits and guidelines for persons with diabetes. In *Handbook of Diabetes Medical Nutrition Therapy.* Powers MA, Ed. Gaithersburg, MD, Aspen Publishers, Inc.,1996, pp. 107–129

144. Ruderman N, Devlin JT, Schneider SH, Kriska A (Eds.): *Handbook of Exercise in Diabetes.* Alexandria, VA, American Diabetes Association, 2002

145. Fujioka K: Management of obesity as a chronic disease: nonpharmacologic, pharmacologic, and surgical option. *Obes Res* 10:116S–123S, 2002

146. McGuire MT, Wing RR, Klem ML, Seagle HM, Hill JO: Long-term maintenance of weight loss: do people who lose weight through various weight loss methods use different

behaviors to maintain their weight? *Int J Obes* 22:572–577, 1998

147. American Diabetes Association: Physical activity/exercise and diabetes mellitus (Position Statement). *Diabetes Care* 26 (Suppl. 1):S73–77, 2003

148. Schneider SH, Shindler D: Application of the American Diabetes Association's guidelines for the evaluation of the diabetic patient before recommending an exercise program. In *Handbook of Exercise in Diabetes*. Ruderman N, Devlin JT, Schneider SH, Kriska A (Eds.) Alexandria, VA, American Diabetes Association, 2002

149. Dahlkoetter J, Callahan EJ, Linton J: Obesity and the unbalanced energy equation: exercise versus eating habit change. *J Consult Clin Psychol* 47: 898–905, 1979

150. Bouchard C, Depres JP, Tremblay A: Exercise and obesity. *Obesity Res* 1:133–147, 1993

151. Pate RR, Pratt M, Blair SN, Haskell WL, Macera CA, Bouchard C, Buchner D, Ettinger W, Heath GW, King AC: Physical activity and public health: a recommendation from the Centers for Disease Control and prevention and the American College of Sports Medicine. *JAMA* 273: 402–407, 1995

152. Jakicic JM, Winters C, Lang W, Wing RR: Effects of intermittent exercise and use of home exercise equipment on adherence, weight loss, and fitness in overweight women: a randomized trial. *JAMA* 282:1554–1560, 1999

153. Lee DC, Blair SN, Jackson AS: Cardiorespiratory fitness, body composition, and all-cause and cardiovascular disease mortality in men. *Am J Clin Nutr* 69:373–380, 1999

154. Farrell SW, Braun LA, Barlow CE, Cheng YJ, Blair SN: The relation of body mass index, cardiorespiratory fitness, and all-cause mortality in women. *Obesity Research* 10:417–423, 2002

155. Wei M, Gibbons LW, Kampert JB, Nichaman MZ, Blair SN: Low cardiorespiratory fitness and physical inactivity as predictors of mortality in men with type 2 diabetes. *Ann Intern Med* 132:605–611, 2000

156. Wei M, Gibbons LW, Mitchell TL, Kampert JB, Lee CD, Blair SN: The association between cardiorespiratory fit-

ness and impaired fasting glucose and type 2 diabetes in men. *Ann Intern Med* 130:89–96, 1999

157. Duncan GE, Perri MG, Theriaque DW, Hutson Ad, Eckel RH, Stacpoole PW: Exercise training, without weight loss, increases insulin sensitivity and postheparin, plasma lipase activity in previously sedentary adults. *Diabetes Care* 26:557–562, 2003

158. Landrum S: *Small Steps Big Rewards: Walking Your Way to Better Health* (book and pedometer). Alexandria, VA, Small Steps Press, 2003

159. White JR, Campbell RK: Pharmacologic therapies for glucose management. In *Diabetes Management Therapies. A CORE Curriculum for Diabetes Education.* 5th ed. Franz MJ, Ed. Chicago, American Association of Diabetes Educators, 2003, pp. 95–151

160. Bolderman KM: *Putting Your Patients on the Pump.* Alexandria, VA, American Diabetes Association, 2002

161. Hinnen DA, Guthrie DW, Childs BP, Friesen J, Rhiley DS, Guthrie RA: Pattern management of blood glucose. In *A CORE Curriculum for Diabetes: Diabetes Management Therapies.* 5th ed. Franz M, Ed. Chicago, American Association of Diabetes Educators, 2003, p. 213–246

162. USDA Center for Nutrition Policy and Promotion: Eating breakfast greatly improves schoolchildren's diet quality. *Nutrition Insights* 15: Dec 1999, http://www.usda.gov/cnpp/insights.html (accessed September 2, 2003)

163. Reuters Health Information: Eating breakfast may stave off obesity, diabetes. Reuters Limited, http://www.heartcenteronline.com/myheartdr/home/researchdetail.cfm?reutersid=3434 (accessed September 2, 2003)

164. Arnold L, Mann JI, Ball MJ: Metabolic effects of alterations in meal frequency in type 2 diabetes. *Diabetes Care* 20:1151–1154, 1997

165. Dwyer JT, Evans M, Stone EJ, Feldman HA, Lytle L, Hoelscher D, Johnson C, Zive M, Yang M: Adolescents' eating patterns influence their nutrient intakes. *J Am Diet Assoc* 101:798–802, 2001

166. Pearson J, Bergenstal R: Fine-tuning control: pattern management versus supplementation. *Diabetes Spectrum* 14:75–78, 2001

167. Hirsch IR, Farkas-Hirsh R: Sliding scale or sliding scare: it's all sliding nonsense. *Diabetes Spectrum* 14:79–81, 2001

168. American Diabetes Association: *Intensive Diabetes Management.* 3rd ed. Klingensmith GK, Ed. Alexandria, VA, American Diabetes Association, 2003

169. Taubes G: What if it's all been a big fat lie? *New York Times,* 7 July 2002: New York Times Magazine, pp. 22–27, 34–36

170. Liebman B: The truth about the Atkins diet. *Nutrition Action* 29:1–7, 2002

171. Neville K: Are low fat diets really a big fat lie? EN weighs in. *Environmental Nutrition* 25:1, Oct 2002

172. Foster GD, Wyatt HR, Hill JO, McGuckin BG, Brill D, Mohammed S, Szapary PO, Rader DJ, Edman JS, Klein S. A randomized trial of a low-carbohydrate for obesity. *N Engl J Med* 348(21) 2082-2090. 2003

173. Bravata DM, Sanders L, Kuang J, Krumholz HM, Olkin I, Gardner CD, Bravata D: Efficacy and safety of low-carbohydrate diets: a systematic review. *JAMA* 289:1837–1850, 2003

174. North American Association for the Study of Obesity: Popular diets: a scientific review. *Obes Res* 9 (Suppl. 1):1S–40S, 2001

175. Anderson JW, Konz E, Jenkins D: Health advantages and disadvantages of weight reducing diets: a computer analysis and critical review. *J Am Clin Nutr* 19:578–590, 2000

176. Rock C: A view on high-protein, low-carb diets. *J Am Diet Assoc* 100:1300–1302, 2000

177. Reddy ST: Low carb diets tax kidneys. *Am J Kidney Dis* 40:265–274, 2002

178. World Health Organization: Obesity: preventing and managing the global epidemic. Report of the World Health Organization Consultation on Obesity. June 3–5, 1997, Geneva, Switzerland, World Health Organization, 1998

179. Zhu S, Wang Z, Heksa S, Moonseong H, Faith MS, Heymsfield SB: Waist circumference and obesity-associated risk factors among white in the third National

Health and Nutrition Examination Survey: clinical action thresholds. *Am J Clin Nutr* 76:743–749, 2002

180. Klem ML, Wing RR, McGuire MT, Seagle HM, Hill JO: A descriptive study of individuals successful with long-term maintenance of substantial weight loss. *Am J Clin Nutr* 66:239–246, 1997

181. Schick SM, Wing RR, Klem ML, McGuire J, Hill J, Seagle H: People successful at long-term weight loss and maintenance continue to consume a low-energy, low-fat diet. *J Am Diet Ass* 98:408–413, 1998

182. Wyatt H, Grunwald GK, Mosca CL, Klem ML, Wing RR, Hill JO: Long-term weight loss and breakfast in subjects in the National Weight Control Registry. *Obes Res* 10:78–82, 2002

183. McGuire MT, Wing RR, Klem ML, Seagle HM, Hill JO: Long-term maintenance of weight loss: do people who lose weight through various weight loss methods use different behaviors to maintain their weight? *Int J Obes* 22:572–577, 1998

184. Klem ML, Wing RR, Ho Chang CC, Lang W, McGuire MT, Sugerman HJ, Hutchinson SL, Makovich AL, Hill JO: A case-control study of successful maintenance of a substantial weight loss: individuals who lost weight through surgery versus those who lost weight through non-surgical means. *Int J Obes* 24:573–579, 2000

185. Institute of Medicine: *Weighing the Options: Criteria for Evaluation Weight Management Programs.* Washington, DC, National Academy Press, 1995

186. Knowler WC, Barrett-Connor E, Fowler SE, Hamman RF, Lachin JM, Walked EA, Nathan DM: Reduction in the incidence of type 2 diabetes with lifestyle intervention or metformin. *N Engl J Med* 346:393–403, 2002

187. Dixon JB, O'Brien PE: Health outcomes of severly obese type 2 diabetic subjects 1 year after laparoscopic adjustable gastric banding. *Diabetes Care* 25:358–363, 2002

188. Brolin RD: Bariatric surgery and long-term control of morbid obesity. *JAMA* 288:2793–2796, 2002

189. Dymek MP, LeGrange D, Neven K, Alverdy J: Quality of life after gastric bypass surgery: a cross-sectional study. *Obes Res* 10:1135–1142, 2002

190. Lustman PJ, Griffith LS, Clouse RE: Recognizing and managing depression in patients with diabetes. In *Practical Psychology for the Diabetes Clinician*. Anderson BJ, Rubin RR, Eds. Alexandria, VA, American Diabetes Association, 2022, pp. 229–238

191. Polonsky WH, Parkin CG: Depression in patients with diabetes: seven facts every health-care provider should know. *Practical Diabetology* December 20–29, 2001

192. Edege LE, Zheng D, Simpson K : Comorbid depression is associated with increased health care use in individuals with diabetes. *Diabetes Care* 25:464–470, 2002

193. Nettles AT: Diabetes in older adults. In *Diabetes in the Life Cycle and Research. A CORE Curriculum for Diabetes Educators*. 5th ed. Franz MJ, Ed. Chicago, American Association of Diabetes Educators, 2003, pp. 179–201

194. Funnell MM, Arnold MS, Fogler J, Merritt JH, Anderson LA: Participation in a diabetes education and care program: experience from the diabetes care for older adults project. *Diabetes Educator* 24:163–167, 1998

195. American Diabetes Association: Gestational diabetes (Position Statement). *Diabetes Care* 25 (Suppl. 1):S103–105, 2003

196. Biastre SA, Slocum J: Gestational diabetes. In *Diabetes in the Life Cycle and Research. A CORE Curriculum for Diabetes Educators*. 5th ed. Franz MJ, Ed. Chicago, American Association of Diabetes Educators, 2003, pp. 145–173

197. Warshaw HS: *Eat Out, Eat Right*. Chicago, Surrey Books, 2003

198. Warshaw HS: *Guide to Healthy Restaurant Eating*. 2nd ed. Alexandria, VA, American Diabetes Association, 2002

199. Umpierrez GE, Murphy MB, Kitabchi AE: Diabetic ketoacidosis and hyperglycemic hyperosmolar syndrome. *Diabetes Spectrum* 15:28–36, 2002

200. American Diabetes Association: Hyperglycemic crises in patients with diabetes mellitus (Position Statement). *Diabetes Care* 26 (Suppl. 1):S109–117, 2003

201. Cryer PE, Childs BP: Negotiating the barrier of hypoglycemia in diabetes mellitus. *Diabetes Spectrum* 15:20–27, 2002

202. Schafer R, Bohannon B, Franz MJ, Freeman J, Holmes A, McLaughlin S, Haas L, Kruger D, Lorenz R, McMahon M: Translation of the diabetes nutrition recommendtion for health care institutions (Technical Review). *Diabetes Care* 20:96–105, 1997

203. White J, Davis S, Cooppan R, Davidson MB, Mulcahy K, Manko G, Nelinson D: Clarifying the role of insulin in type 2 diabetes management. *Clinical Diabetes* 21:14–21, 2003

204. Ohkubo Y, Kishikawa H, Araki E, Miyata T, Isami S, Motoyoshi S, Kojima Y, Furuyoshi N, Shichiri M: Intensive insulin therapy prevents the progression of diabetic microvasuclar complication in Japanese patients with non-insulin-dependent diabetes: a reandomized propsepctive 6 year study. *Diabetes Res Clin Pract* 28:103–117, 1995

205. Cryer PE, Fisher JN, Shamoon H: Hypoglycemia (Technical Review). *Diabetes Care* 17:734–755, 1994

206. Brodows RG, Williams C, Amatruda JM: Treatment of insulin reactions in diabetics. *JAMA* 252:3378–3381, 1984

207. Slama G, Traynard P-Y, Desplanque N, Pudar H, Dhunputh I, Letanoux M, Bornet FRJ, Tchobroutsky G: The search for an optimized treatment of hypoglycemia. *Arch Intern Med* 150:589–593, 1990

208. Schvarcz E, Palmaer M, Aman J, Lindkvist B, Beckman K-W: Hypoglycemia increases gastric emptying rate in patients with type 1 diabetes mellitus. *Diabetic Med* 10:660–663, 1993

209. Gray RO, Butler PC, Beers TR, Kryshak EJ, Rizza RA: Comparison of the ability of bread versus bread plus meat to treat and prevent subsequent hypoglycemia in patients with insulin-dependent diabetes mellitus. *J Clin Endocrinol Metab* 81:1508–1511, 1996

210. Neilson SJ, Popkin BM: Patterns and trends in food portion sizes, 1977–1998. *JAMA* 289:450–453, 2003

211. Young LR, Nestle M: Expanding portion sizes in the U.S. marketplace: implications for nutrition counseling. *J Am Diet Assoc* 103:231–234, 2003

212. Jenkins DJA, Ocana A, Jenkins AL, Wolever TMS, Vuksan V, Katzman L, Hollands M, Greenberg G, Corey P, Patten R, Wong G, Josse RG: Metabolic advantages of spreading the nutrient load: effects of increased meal frequency in non-insulin-dependent diabetes. *Am J Clin Nutr* 55:461–467, 1992

213. Bertelsen J, Christiansen C, Thomsen C, Poulsen PL, Vestergaard S, Steinov A, Rasmussen LH, Rasmussen O, Hermansen K: Effect of meal frequency on blood glucose, insulin, and free fatty acids in NIDDM subject. *Diabetes Care* 16:4–7, 1993

214. Beebe CA, Van Cauter E, Shapiro T, Tillel H, Lyons R, Rubenstein A, Polonsky K: Effects of temporal distribution of calories on diurnal patterns of glucose levels and insulin secretion in NIDDM. *Diabetes Care* 13:748–755, 1990

215. Kalergis M, Schiffrin A, Gougeon R, Jone PJH, Yale J-F: Impact of bedtime snack composition on prevention of nocturnal hypoglycemia in adults with type 1 diabetes undergoing intensive insulin managment using lispro insulin before meals: a randomized, placebo-controlled, crossover trial. *Diabetes Care* 26:9–15, 2003

216. Mokdad AH, Bowman BA, Ford ES, Vinicor F, Marks JS, Koplan JP: The continuing epidemics of obesity and diabetes in the United States. *JAMA* 12:1195–1200, 2001

217. Delahanty, L: Evidence-Based trends for achieving weight loss and increased physical activity: applications for diabetes prevention and treatment. *Diabetes Spectrum* 15: 183–189, 2002

218. American Diabetes Association, National Institute of Diabetes, Digestive and Kidney Diseases: The prevention or delay of type 2 diabetes (Position Statement). *Diabetes Care* 25:742–749, 2002

219. The Diabetes Prevention Program (DPP) Research Group: The Diabetes Prevention Program: description of lifestyle intervention. *Diabetes Care* 25:2165–2171, 2002

220. The Center for Weight and Health, University of California at Berkeley: Prevention of childhood over-weight—what should be done? (Position Paper). Center for Weight and Health, University of California at Berkeley, http://nature.berkeley.edu/cwh/activities/position.shtml (accessed August 28, 2003)

221. Vickery L: Don't supersize it—and other tips for parents working to mend their kids' junk-food ways. *The Wall Street Journal.* 11 Nov 2002: Sect. R, p.10

222. Satter E: *How to Get Your Kids to Eat But Not Too Much.* Palo Alto, CA, Bull Human Kinetics, 1996

223. Centers for Disease Control and Prevention: Prevalence of overweight among children and adolescents: United States, 1999–2000. Centers for Disease Control and Prevention, http://www.cdc.gov/nchs/products/pubs/pubd/hestats/overwght99.htm (accessed August 28, 2003)

224. Reader D, Sipe M: Key components of care for women with gestational diabetes. *Diabetes Spectrum* 14:188–191, 2001

225. American Diabetes Association: Government relations and advocacy. American Diabetes Association, http://www.diabetes.org/main/community/advocacy/default.jsp (accessed September 2, 2003)

226. American Diabetes Association: Part B Medicare benefits for medical nutrition therapy (MNT): a web-based resource. American Diabetes Association, http://www.diabetes.org/main/professional/recognition/default.jsp (accessed September 2, 2003)

227. American Association of Diabetes Educators: Part B Medicare benefits for MNT for diabetes and renal disease. American Association of Diabetes Educators, http://www.aadenet.org/Advocacy/ReimburseResources/MNTIndex.html (accessed September 2, 2003)

228. American Dietetic Association: Medical nutrition therapy (MNT) services available to Medicare patients. American

Dietetic Association, http://www.eatright.org/Public/GovernmentAffairs/98_12461.cfm (accessed September 2, 2003)

229. American Dietetic Association's Diabetes Care and Education Practice Group: Part B Medicare benefits for MNT for diabetes and renal disease: a web based resource. American Dietetic Association, http://www.dce.org/homepage/MNTbenefit.htm (accessed September 2, 2003)

230. Monk A, Barry B, McClain K, Weaver T, Cooper M, Franz MJ: Practice guidelines for medical nutrition therapy by dietitians for people with non-insulin-dependent diabetes mellitus. *J Am Diet Assoc* 95:999–1008, 1995

231. Diabetes Care and Education Practice Group of the American Dietetic Association: *Diabetes Nutrition Practice Guidelines Pocket Guide: A Companion Resource to the American Dietetic Association MNT Evidence Based Guides for Practice.* Chicago, American Dietetic Association, 2002

232. Warshaw H, Bourgeois P, Postigo C (Eds.): *The Guide to Reimbursement.* Chicago, American Association of Diabetes Educators, 2003, p.109

233. Feste CC: *Empowerment: Facilitating a Path to Personal Self-Care.* Elkart, IN, Miles, 1991

234. Tunis S, Phurrough S, Stojak M, Chin J, Ulrich M: Decision memo: duration and frequency of the medical nutrition therapy (MNT) benefit (#CAG-00097N). Centers for Medicare and Medicaid Services, http://63.241.27.78/mcd/viewdecisionmemo.asp?id=53 (accessed September 2, 2003)

235. Ford E, Giles W, Dietz W: Prevalence of the metabolic syndrome among US adults. *JAMA* 287:356–359, 2002

236. Practice Management Information Corporation (PMIC): *International Classification of Diseases.* 9th ed. Los Angeles, Practice Management Information Corporation, 2003

237. Urbanski P: Reimbursement strategies for pre-diabetes. *On the Cutting Edge* 23:37–39, 2002

238. Fitzner K, Myers E, Caputo N, Michael P: Are health plans changing their view on nutrition service coverage? *J Am Diet Assoc* 103:157–161, 2003

About the American Diabetes Association

The American Diabetes Association is the nation's leading voluntary health organization supporting diabetes research, information, and advocacy. Its mission is to prevent and cure diabetes and to improve the lives of all people affected by diabetes. The American Diabetes Association is the leading publisher of comprehensive diabetes information. Its huge library of practical and authoritative books for people with diabetes covers every aspect of self-care—cooking and nutrition, fitness, weight control, medications, complications, emotional issues, and general self-care.

To order American Diabetes Association books:
Call 1-800-232-6733. Or log on to http://store.diabetes.org

To join the American Diabetes Association: Call 1-800-806-7801.
www.diabetes.org/membership

For more information about diabetes or ADA programs and services:
Call 1-800-342-2383.
E-mail: Customerservice@diabetes.org or log on to www.diabetes.org

To locate an ADA/NCQA Recognized Provider of quality diabetes care in your area: www.ncqa.org/dprp

To find an ADA Recognized Education Program in your area: Call 1-888-232-0822.
www.diabetes.org/recognition/education.asp

To join the fight to increase funding for diabetes research, end discrimination, and improve insurance coverage:
Call 1-800-342-2383. www.diabetes.org/advocacy

To find out how you can get involved with the programs in your community:
Call 1-800-342-2383. See below for program Internet addresses.

- *American Diabetes Month:* Educational activities aimed at those diagnosed with diabetes—month of November. www.diabetes.org/ADM
- *American Diabetes Alert:* Annual public awareness campaign to find the undiagnosed—held the fourth Tuesday in March. www.diabetes.org/alert
- *The Diabetes Assistance & Resources Program (DAR):* Diabetes awareness program targeted to the Latino community. www.diabetes.org/DAR
- *African American Program:* Diabetes awareness program targeted to the African American community. www.diabetes.org/africanamerican
- *Awakening the Spirit: Pathways to Diabetes Prevention & Control:* Diabetes awareness program targeted to the Native American community. www.diabetes.org/awakening

To find out about an important research project regarding type 2 diabetes:
www.diabetes.org/ada/research.asp

To obtain information on making a planned gift or charitable bequest:
Call 1-888-700-7029. www.diabetes.org/ada/plan.asp

To make a donation or memorial contribution:
Call 1-800-342-2383. www.diabetes.org/ada/cont.asp